making a way

PRAISE FOR *MAKING A WAY*

"This book is for anyone along the Medical Medium spectrum, from wide-eyed newbies to the most seasoned practitioners.

"Deborah concisely summarizes Medical Medium information and offers her insights. Even as someone deeply embedded in this world, I found myself struck by details I had forgotten or long since glanced over; it's a rare find that manages to simplify the complex while still delivering fresh aha! moments for the experts.

"Deborah's story is the perfect vehicle to show how one can surmount health challenges while navigating naysaying loved ones and the friction of the modern world. In the end, this book is more than just a guide; it is a steady hand on your shoulder. It proves that even in the face of daunting adversity, the path to healing remains open, providing the clarity needed to refine your protocols and the unwavering faith necessary to navigate the toughest stretches of the journey."

—Nguyen Phan, MD

making
a way

RISING FROM CHRONIC PAIN, ILLNESS, AND LYME DISEASE

Deborah Kelly

with an afterword by John Kelly

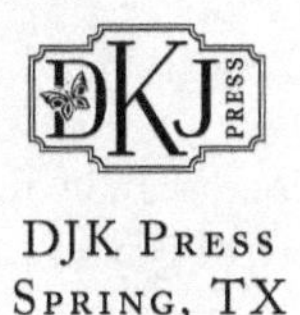

DJK Press
Spring, TX

DJK Press
Spring, TX

Some names and identifying features or persons have been modified and anonymized to protect confidentiality and privacy.

This memoir reflects the author's personal experiences and is intended for informational purposes only. Nothing in this book should be construed as medical, psychological, or professional advice. The author is not a licensed healthcare provider, and the experiences described are unique to the author's circumstances. Readers should consult qualified healthcare professionals before making any decisions regarding their own medical care, treatment, or lifestyle changes. The author and publisher disclaim any liability for adverse effects resulting from the use or application of the information contained in this book.

Library of Congress Control Number: 2026908493

Paperback ISBN: 979-8-9941843-0-1
eBook ISBN: 979-8-9941843-1-8

Book cover design and interior design by Erin Seaward-Hiatt
Author photo by Karina Eremina (joyofthemomentphotography.com)
Editorial production by KN Literary Arts

For those looking for a way to truly heal emotionally, mentally, physically, and spiritually.

Contents

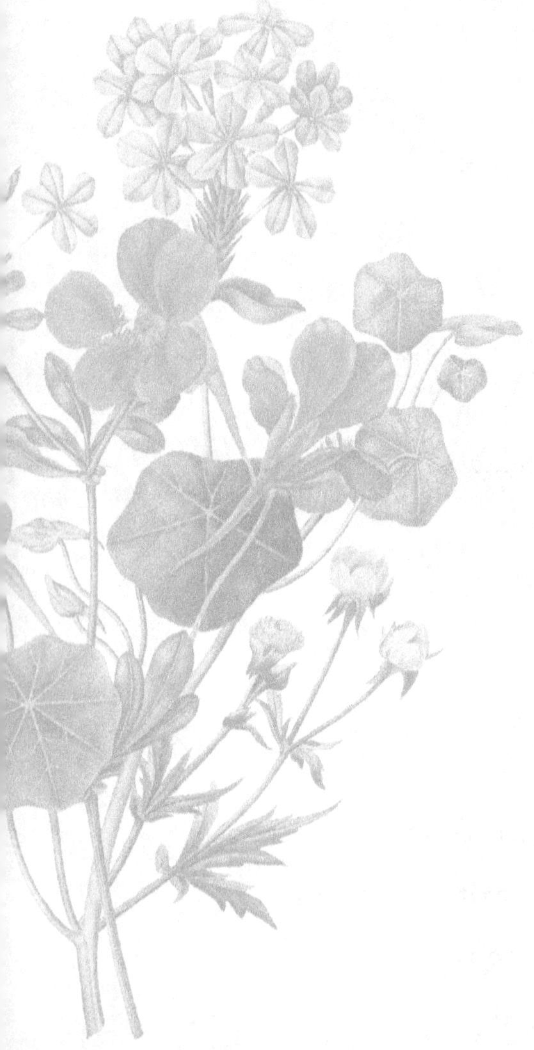

Preface

Insomnia had set in, even though the fatigue was relentless. The accident left me with more pain than I knew how to handle. One night, when everyone else was asleep, I walked into the living room and sat under a blanket in a recliner between the TV and the window. I had nowhere else to go. I looked up and had a desperate conversation.

"God, what is this pain all about? I can't live with this pain for the rest of my life. I don't know what You want me to do with this. I'm only forty-one years old. I don't want to be on pain medication for the rest of my life, and I don't want to become an addict."

In the darkness and stillness, I sensed an unmistakable message, encompassing me with a familiar power.

This is not about you; it is bigger than you. Write a book.

"Did I just hear that?" I wondered. Yes, I'd heard it but not with my ears—I had felt it.

"I have three children, a husband, and a dog all counting on me, and you want me to write a book?" I waited, but the crisp message hung in the air without further dialogue. I didn't expect it. The pain I was having very much felt "all about me!" It didn't feel bigger than me, and I was a mom, not a writer.

But my mom had always taught me to learn a lesson from each experience, whether positive or negative. I knew there had to be purpose to the pain, so I began to journal. I typed notes on my phone with my left thumb, since I couldn't use my right hand. Years later, I emailed those notes to myself and had them bound into journals. I had no idea then what I was going to find; I just knew there was *more* out there. Indeed, there was so much more than I could imagine.

CHAPTER 1

SOS

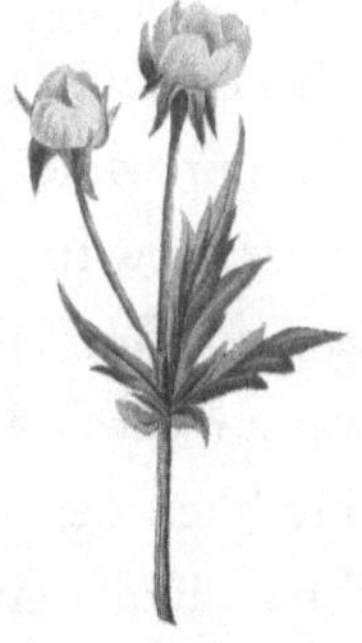

"DINNER'S READY!" I CALLED out to the kids. Patrick had just been dropped off from football practice. Using his long and lean tanned legs, he ran upstairs like a gazelle into his navy-blue room, where he laid his backpack and trombone in their usual spot. Always hungry as an eighth grader at the local junior high, he was eager to eat anything.

"Can you set the table, please?" I asked.

"Yes, sure, I'm starving, and I have a lot to do tonight," he commented. "Tomorrow, I have an algebra test, I've got to practice my trombone because I have a chair test on Friday, and I have a history project due soon."

"I'm sure you will get everything done," I encouraged. He had a knack for being a go-getter like me, and he had my dark eyes and dark curly hair. His fourth-grade teacher had valued his quick wit, telling me it was a sign of intelligence. As our oldest child at fifteen years of age, Patrick was diligent, followed the rules, and had thrived on a schedule since birth, always wanting to know what was next, like his dad. He drew people in with his hospitality, loving a crowd and a plan, and being involved just like his mom. His warm, kind smile was always intact amid his abs of steel.

The aroma from the beef stew in the crockpot and the rice on the stove carried from our white gourmet kitchen, up the rich cherry-stained stairs. It drew thirteen-year-old Evan away from his game of Mario Kart. Beef stew was a family favorite, but Evan particularly was a meat-and-potatoes kid and hardly an adventurous eater. He liked dependability, and instead of eagerly jumping into things like a swimming pool before he knew how to swim, he was a cautious teenager in our new home. His broad shoulders and muscular calves, along with his deep brownish-green puppy dog eyes, only added to his charisma. His sixth-grade homeroom teacher once told me he was just like a friendly yellow Labrador retriever, easy-going, smart, and energetic. He even had the same coloring as a lab, with his dirty blonde hair amid red tones and fair skin like his Irish dad.

"Can someone please fill the glasses with water?" I asked.

"Sarah's got it," Evan quickly answered, the ever-ready delegator.

"Where is Sarah?" I wondered, then immediately caught her red-handed in the pantry, holding a bag of Goldfish crackers. "I told you, NO snacking before dinner!" I said on repeat, for the millionth time. Sarah showed her silly side, shimmying her seven-year-old, second-grade self out of the pantry over to pet our dog Fluffy, perched on the back of the couch. When she was a toddler, strangers would stop and comment on Sarah's radiant beauty. My high-school English teacher would have recited Keats when describing Sarah as "a thing of beauty is a joy forever." I often thought she made her brothers look more alike, as she had Evan's hair color and Patrick's stature and trim figure, combined with her own bluish-greenish eyes and medium skin tone. It was her third-grade teacher who assured me she was a wiz in math, was the fastest on the playground, enjoyed reading, and was a pleasure in the classroom, yet preferred to be inconspicuous. As her mom, I focused on her inner beauty and caring nature.

Fluffy was our ten-pound Havanese. She was dark gray and a sweet, furry friend to everyone. She exuded unconditional love and kindness to our family, to strangers, and to other dogs when we went for hikes on the neighborhood walking trails. Not a lap dog but always wanting to be near her human, she followed me around the house like my shadow. My athletic boys named her Fluffy Angel Kelly when they were young. But that's exactly what she was—our fluffy angel.

"Evan and Sarah, fill the water glasses together," I instructed. My husband, John, had texted he'd left the office about an hour ago and would walk in the door at any moment. He used the hour commute to transform from his Houston petroleum engineer executive self back to a calm suburban dad and husband. His hair was becoming slightly salt-and-peppered, changing from the light-brown MacGyver look he used to have. His eyes gleamed with blue-green hazel chameleon vibes like Sarah's, altering as they changed their wardrobes. Always a critical thinker and analyzer, John kept many of his own thoughts to himself. One of his top strengths was being able to see things from multiple points of view. An avid reader with incredible retention, John would be the perfect phone-a-friend. He was the kind of dad who didn't bring his work home. Often, I'd encourage him to discuss his job so our kids could learn the ins and outs of the corporate world. My dad ran a music store and was on several boards in my hometown, an hour outside of New Orleans, Louisiana. I only knew a fraction about his work environment and hoped our children would learn more, but John was good at the work-life balance.

I, on the other hand, didn't want to miss anything and wanted to do everything. I enjoyed exercising leadership and organizational skills at the kids' schools, working out, and keeping order as a homemaker managing all the moving parts of our family. For me, there wasn't enough time in the day to check off my to-do list. Simplicity wasn't in my nature. As I've always said, John brought balance to my eager-beaver attitude.

When he entered our newly painted two-story southern home dressed in loafers, khakis, and a buttoned-down collared shirt, Fluffy began her normal wild greeting: barking with delight, wagging her tail at one hundred miles per hour, and licking John's hands a few times as he petted her. I received my "I'm home" kiss on the cheek as he unwound from a day's work and then served side salads for everyone.

Each night, we took turns saying a prayer around our wide rectangular dinner table. We gathered in the dining area of the living space, with its raised ceilings overlooking the backyard pool through the windows.

"Thank you for this day and this meal and for all of our blessings. Keep us safe and on the right path," spoke John, our in-house safety expert.

"Hey Mom, pass the GB," blurted Evan.

"Excuse me?" I questioned.

"The GB, you know, the garlic bread," Evan chuckled.

"How was everyone's day?" John asked.

"Fine," the trio synchronized.

"I heard on talk radio that it was better to ask your kids what the best and worst part of their day has been," John remarked, shifting the conversation.

Patrick started, "The best part of my day was basketball tryouts this morning. The worst was I couldn't get my locker opened and had to go to the front office. Mom, dinner is stew-pendous!" he exclaimed and smiled.

"I don't know what my worst was, but my best was playing with Carli on the playground," offered Sarah. "Oh wait, I know what my worst was. Mom said I couldn't have ice cream after school."

"Sarah, you can't have ice cream every day," corrected Evan. "My worst was the bus driver kept yelling at us to sit down, but the best was when Jason snuck under the teacher's desk and tickled her toes. It was hilarious!" he snickered.

I added mine. "My best was having lunch with the second-grade room moms after getting the stew in the crockpot. I really didn't have a worst moment, unless you count bringing Fluffy to the groomer and watching her nervously shake in the car, poor thing.

John, what about you?" I asked, as I took chocolate chip cookies out of the oven for dessert.

"The best part of my day was that our quarterly meetings moved in a positive direction, and it's almost Friday. The worst was missing you guys today. I'm glad to be home."

John and I met when we were both eighteen years old in the middle of our freshman year in college at Louisiana State University. We met at a fraternity/sorority exchange party. I had no plans to stay at this party, but my friend didn't want to leave. My trigonometry test result the next day was a downer. But the upside was I met Mr. FTD (Florist Transworld Delivery)—a nickname given to him by his mom because John courted me with one bouquet of flowers after another. We became best friends and dated for six years, finishing college before getting married. We grew into adulthood together. We began our circle of life as we danced to Elton John's "Can You Feel the Love Tonight" at our wedding. John's engineering job took us to Houston, Texas, away from family and friends in Louisiana.

While in nursing school, I worked at the Manning Family's Children's Hospital (formerly the Children's Hospital of New Orleans) on the hematology/oncology floor. I was anxious to begin working at a major cancer hospital in the Houston Medical Center, where I was assigned to the adolescent unit. We served patients from all over the world with osteosarcoma, lymphoma, leukemia (which often led to bone marrow transplants), and an assorted array of other diagnoses. On the other end of the unit, we cared for patients who were post-op from mastectomies, prostate surgeries, and other surgeries. They would spend the night on our floor and then be discharged the next day. It was a revolving door on the surgical side, but the same adolescents returned frequently for treatment on the medical side.

Oh, how I wanted to save them all! I hated seeing patients suffering day in and day out. It saddened me to watch the children and their families spending so much time—days, weeks, years—receiving treatment and extracted from their normal lives. It was our job to administer chemotherapy, blood transfusions, medications for nausea and pain, and experimental medications. It was a grind for both our patients and their families. I tried to be kind and supportive, occasionally dancing in with their chemo treatments—anything to get them to smile.

My next job was working in the clinic as the nurse coordinator for patients with neurofibromatosis (NF) at the same hospital. This group had mostly noncancerous tumors developing in their brain, spinal cord, and nerves. Their tumors were external and/or internal. The doctors studied and compared the patients' annual brain magnetic resonance imaging (MRI) scans and assessed any other needs. I scheduled their appointments and scans as I worked alongside an amazing pediatric neurologist.

Before my husband and I knew it, we were living in a wooded Houston suburb with walking/biking trails and community parks and pools. My banker father-in-law had encouraged us to obtain a mortgage based on one person's salary, knowing we wanted children. We were located far away from family and friends and both commuting long distances, so something needed to give when Patrick was born. I chose not to go back to work at the hospital. My full-time job had changed to being a full-time mom. My nursing career of three years had been short-lived yet was certainly impactful. I had learned what medicine is capable of rectifying, along with its limitations. In addition, I also learned the value of good health.

John was still commuting into the city, and I was CEO of our home and children. Life was good, and it's true that children grow up way too fast. We kept the kids busy with plenty of toys, every imaginable activity and lesson, church classes, and multiple sports. Our lives were full, and we tackled challenges as they came and went. When our children were becoming more independent, I began seeing other moms returning to work—the kind of work with a paycheck to assist with college tuition. I wondered if it was time to find a job besides volunteering in the schools. I turned to God, asking about His purpose and plan for me, then waited for guidance.

On February 21, 2012, I had an accident. It was Mardi Gras day—a day that every town in southern Louisiana celebrates as Fat Tuesday. But now that we lived in Texas, I had only memories of Mardi Gras remaining vivid in my mind. Back home, Mardi Gras was a huge part of our social culture. My dad's music store was on the Mardi Gras parade route in our hometown. We knew many float riders for the multiple parades, so we were guaranteed to walk away with treasures that were thrown by them each time. Our family friends would gather amid the pianos, guitars, and band instruments in the air conditioning as we awaited each parade. There was always a potluck assortment of picnic foods, drinks, fried chicken, and, of course, king cake to be eaten.

My parents were involved with some of the Mardi Gras crews, and each of them rode on a float. When I was young, I was a page to the queen of the Mardi Gras crew and was able to ride in the parade in a convertible. As a teenager, I was a maid to the queen, which involved attending multiple parties and standing at city hall for the parade, dressed in a black-and-white polka-dotted suit and matching hat. My mom was in an all-women's crew, and my dad was in an all-men's crew. I used to go with my mom to the float hall to help the ladies decorate their float. I probably spent more time running around the float warehouse and climbing on and off each float than I did decorating.

That day, I brought those memories and sheer joy onto the tennis court with Mardi Gras beads around my neck. My ponytail, visor, and sunglasses were ready to perform. We called ourselves the Green Machine, hence our matching green tennis skirts. I had played tennis since I was a kid and was on the team in high school, then I joined a league when my kids were in school. Tennis was my exercise and my escape, two mornings a week. On this day, the weather was even cooperating as the sun shone brightly, warming us to a comfortable seventy-five degrees Fahrenheit without clouds or wind.

"Happy Mardi Gras!" I cheered at Kristin, my slim and trim partner for the match. She was always relaxed and had daughters my age.

"Happy Mardi Gras to you! I hope you brought king cake as promised," she replied.

"You know I did, along with a few other treats," I offered. "I'll play backhand if you'll take the forehand side?"

"Sounds good to me. I think we got this," she whispered.

We were paired up against two gray-haired players whom we underestimated. We took the first set easily and were well on our way to finishing the match. Then I lunged for a drop shot in the middle of the second set and fell backward on my hands and bottom. The good news: We won the point. The bad news: I knew this tennis season was over, as both my wrists throbbed.

"I don't know if I should keep playing," I told Kristin. But the season had just started, and I didn't want to quit.

"What if we put some ice chips in your wrist bands? I have a pain pill too, if you'd like it?"

"Okay, sure. Let's do that, and hopefully we'll only have a few more points to play."

Against my better judgment, I kept playing, mostly left-handed. Unfortunately, the match was extended to a third set, and I used every stubborn competitive ounce I had to finish the match with a victory. But was it worth it? I couldn't take my clothes off to shower or use the restroom after our match, and I could barely drive. I arrived home after picking up Sarah from second grade then fainted in front of the fireplace, busting my knee on the brick hearth. Frightened, Sarah ran to the housekeeper, who woke me up and had me call John at work, an hour away.

He came home early and helped me shower before taking me to the emergency room. My X-rays showed a broken bone in my right wrist and a sprained left one. Both wrists and my knee were bandaged heavily, but it was the tetanus shot in my arm that hurt the most. When I limped into the house, Evan turned around in his chair with his eyes in shock, exclaiming, "Mom, you are all jacked up!" My kids were used to me being Supermom.

At the next available appointment, I saw an orthopedist who confirmed the results of my X-rays. We told him that we had plans to take the kids skiing for spring break. He said I could ski but to wrap the cast well and be careful. Really? I didn't think that sounded like good advice. A few hours later, I could no longer bear the crushing cast. It was intolerably way too tight. I went back to the orthopedist's office five times in three days, each time getting a new cast that was still painfully compressing my arm. Finally, the physician assistant explained to the cast specialist how to give my hand more space in the cast. He told him to put on a regular cast, cut it open lengthwise to leave a few inches, then add more layers of cast material. The fifth cast was finally comfortable, so away we went to the ski slopes.

I spent most of the week in the condo, reading and napping. We had friends from home in the area, so we joined them for dinner one evening. I remember being in good spirits, despite the temporary setback. For several weeks, I'd had low-grade fevers, achiness, and fatigue. The doctor's office said these symptoms were from the broken bone, but that didn't make sense to me. A broken bone doesn't usually cause a fever, and a fever usually signifies a sign of infection, but their office dismissed my symptoms. I went through a bottle of Motrin in a month, even though I'm not fond of taking medication, knowing their side effects.

Friends and family members helped with evening meals, transportation, and encouragement. Small daily tasks were difficult because I couldn't use my hands. I couldn't drive a car or open or close the kitchen oven; even personal grooming was a challenge. After a few weeks, I could use my left hand, but simple tasks remained difficult, and any email I sent was typed one-handed, without capital letters. I relied on much help planning the sixth-grade field trip and pitching in for the elementary parent-teacher organization fundraiser, as I was PTO president that year. Because I couldn't dry or style my hair, much less apply makeup, I had my hair and makeup done for the fundraiser so I would look more like my usual self.

John's mom, Frannie, was in town, visiting and helping us. She was an avid reader and knew her way around her laptop. Her nickname when her boys were young was the Hawk, because she had a way of sleuthing information. Frannie said her friend's husband once coined her the swizzle stick in the cocktail. She was always easy to spot, tastefully bedazzled with gold and gemstone jewelry that would only be too big on someone else. A Cajun-flared Southern belle dressed to the nines, she didn't leave home without her hair in place, and red "pipstick" on her lips matching her Aunt Pip's lipstick.

She continues to be an expert in simplifying, baking cakes, and taking part in creative outlets like flower arranging and needlepointing. She adores all beautiful things, such as fine fabric, rich decor, and an elegant white rose. Once she saw my predicament, she had a frank conversation with me about getting more help before she returned home. She asked how I planned to feed my family once the meal train ended. I immediately thought about Amber—a mom I knew from the PTO who was a personal chef. I hired her right away, and she began cooking three meals a week for my family every Monday.

I thought needing so much help would be temporary. I was told my right hand would be in a cast for a couple of weeks and braced for a few more, then I would be back to my normal routine. However, the cast remained on for four weeks before my wrist was braced. One night, I was having trouble taking off the removable brace. My fingers were immovable, so I forced the brace with harsh tugs until my slight thumb movement produced excruciating crushing pain.

I began running around, screaming in horrific pain, while John looked at me as if I were out of my mind. It felt as if I had slammed my hand in a car door. I ran from my bathroom to the bedroom, then into the openness of the living room. I bypassed the kitchen and the dining room, going into the study. I kept repeating this lap. I don't know why I ran; I just ran, perhaps hoping to release the pain as I went. I'd never felt pain like that before, and I'd given birth to three children without any epidurals.

I was supposed to be able to take the brace on and off, as needed. The pain was too great for me, however, to remove the brace again, and I was told to simply leave it on and return to the doctor's office in four weeks. After two weeks in the brace, I could not move my right hand at all. My entire hand and wrist were stuck in a clawlike position. The brace remained on until I could get in to see the same orthopedist. I had to wait until after the long Easter holiday weekend, even though I had explained to the doctor's office that my hand and wrist were frozen and my fingers were completely unmovable.

My mom, Millie, was in town helping us then, so she drove me to my appointment. Millie was also a Southern belle but had ditched the hair color and embraced graying naturally. She was always adorned in full makeup and pink lipstick when she left the house or had company coming, as she was a natural hostess who always displayed cheery seasonal decor. At home she had her father's green thumb, always playing in her garden. She still adores a variety of flowers and plants, yet the whimsical daisy remains her favorite flower. She had modeled for Delta Airlines back in the day, when she lived in the French Quarter and had been a flight attendant. She swore she would find all the best bakeries wherever she landed to satisfy her sweet tooth. A spiritual guru at heart, she was always seeking higher guidance. She keeps busy now doing water aerobics and playing dominoes with her friends, while staying creative with sketching and painting. Millie demonstrated being an engaged stay-at-home mother who disciplined my brother and me while also making us feel safe and loved. I inherited her hospitable nature and love of tennis.

My wrist was X-rayed with the brace on, and then the brace was sawed off my hand, as if it were a cast. After I saw the doctor and he assessed my hand's immobility, many workers began coming in and out of my room. It was unusual! They walked in, looked at me and my hand, then walked out. The physician assistant mumbled the letters "RSD" under his breath. As a nurse, I'd been on the other side, assessing a strange problem with a patient, so I recognized the hysteria.

Oh my God, this isn't good! This is more of a problem than I anticipated, I thought, as alarm bells rang in my head. Suddenly, the doctor came back in the room, stating my bone had been healed "completely," but that my body was responding awkwardly to the situation. He said the nurse would be in with further instructions. Then I watched the back of his white lab coat as he briskly walked away from me, down the hall and around the corner, leaving me baffled and confused. He had passed me off to the nurse to handle!

The wiry-haired blonde nurse entered the room with instructions that I was to attend a "special" appointment in two hours with a hand therapist located thirty minutes away, and if that didn't work, to return in two days to receive a nerve block. I had never heard of an emergency therapy appointment. I wondered, *Why was this an emergency?* Before I could ask any questions, we were quickly escorted out of the building. My head was spinning, but obediently we drove to the hand appointment. With the therapist's slightest touch to my right hand, I went berserk. The same unbearable pain caused me to erupt into howling screams. I told them I was going to faint, but the therapist showed no signs of concern, while John and Mom's eyes were shocked by my response. It was safe to say the appointment didn't help me, but I wasn't about to return to the neglect and pandemonium of the orthopedist's office. I needed another opinion and was terrified after reading about Reflex Sympathetic Dystrophy (RSD), more recently termed Complex Regional Pain Syndrome (CRPS).

CRPS is ranked as the most painful form of chronic pain known to man by the McGill Pain Index, a pain questionnaire using descriptive words and an intensity scale rather than numerical ratings for pain. The disorder causes lasting burning pain, usually in a limb following surgery, injury, stroke, heart attack, or trauma. The pain is considered out of proportion to the initial injury. The cause is unknown, and there is no cure. CRPS usually affects more women than men. Treatment may include occupational or physical therapy, pain medication, nerve block medications, psychotherapy, and coping strategies. It is common for the pain to spread from limb to limb and potentially to internal organs, leaving people disabled with debilitating neuro-inflammatory symptoms, permanent deformities, and widespread immobility of limbs. It is thought to be underreported and underdiagnosed.

In 2003, experts in the field filed a formal complaint against the American Medical Association (AMA), claiming that the strict eight objective findings required for diagnosing CRPS were actually a reckless assault on patient care. These patients are more likely to respond to early diagnosis and treatment. One physician argued after treating hundreds of patients with CRPS, he could not recall a single case where the patient had all eight objective findings for a diagnosis. Without a medical diagnosis, patients have been denied treatment by their insurance carriers and accused of "faking" their injuries. The 2003 article said, in the advanced stage of the illness, all patients develop psychiatric problems and narcotic dependency and are left incapacitated and often at the mercy of suicide.

I had never heard of this syndrome in nursing school. I hoped the second orthopedist would know what to do.

"I think I have CRPS, and I'm petrified. I can't move my hand or my fingers at all. It's stuck in this claw position. Will I ever be able to use my right hand again? Can you help me? Can you help me heal?" I begged. I knew I was a sight, because my hands were unable to tame the humidity-induced frizzy hair on my head.

Regardless of my presentation, he was reassuring, "Of course, I'll be able to help you!" However, in hindsight, I'm pretty sure he had no idea what he was dealing with and solely concentrated on the care of the broken bone. Upon computed axial tomography (CAT) scan, he found the right wrist to only be forty percent healed instead of "completely" healed as claimed by my first orthopedist. He explained that a scaphoid fracture needed to be cast or splinted while the fracture healed, possibly up to six months, while maintaining full finger movement, which I'd had in the original cast but not in the brace.

"We need to get you back into a splint to protect your wrist. I can't believe your first orthopedist left you unprotected," the doctor explained. He encouraged me to continue seeing the same occupational therapist (OT) and put me back in a splint custom-made by the therapist for my wrist.

After hearing my story, the OT explained how doctors don't get reimbursed much for patient visits and surgery, but they did get reimbursed well for the specialized brace that had turned my hand into a claw. I don't know if there was any truth to his statement, but it would explain the placement of that premature brace. I was in shock, angry, and scared out of my mind, and I didn't know where to turn.

One evening, John walked in the house after work and said with a straightforward look, "I called your second orthopedist's office, asking for confirmation of the CRPS diagnosis, but they said you don't have CRPS."

"What? Let's go outside," I raised my voice and wanted to shield the kids from this conversation. I put down my cellphone and led us out on the patio away from the windows.

Once outside near the fence, I uncharacteristically screamed at John, "What are you doing, calling my doctor? You don't have any medical knowledge. And if I don't have CRPS, then how do you explain the myriad symptoms and extreme pain I'm experiencing?"

"Your doctor said you don't have CRPS!" John retorted, as if his words would make all the pain vanish.

"If I don't have this condition, then what has happened to my deformed hand? Don't you *ever* call my doctor again!" I warned in the heat of the moment, turning to go back inside to gather everyone for dinner. I couldn't believe that he'd called my doctor without consulting me. What was my husband doing? Was anyone on my side? I don't know if a person knows if they are crazy, but I *did* know that I *wasn't* crazy. It became clear that I was in a crazy situation, and I wasn't going to get better answers or more information if I kept visiting different orthopedists. I felt backed into a corner, so I reached out to my contact list with a massive SOS email.

There were a few significant responses. My sister-in-law alerted her brother-in-law, a physiatrist—a special rehabilitation physician trained to treat patients with injuries, disabilities, and pain medicine. I'd known him for many years, but we had never spoken on the phone. He called me right away, emphasizing immediate nerve blocks being the treatment of choice. I was relieved to speak with a familiar person who was educated and treated other patients with this problem, yet I was leery to have an intervention without understanding the cause. CRPS is thought to be caused by a dysfunction in the nervous system. I asked him why this was happening and what was causing the condition. The nurse in me wanted to understand the physiology behind the deformity and pain. He spoke honestly, saying doctors don't know why this happens; it just does. I appreciated him taking the time to share his expertise.

A friend from Evan's preschool days with a nursing background phoned to give me a contact. She had a friend who had this condition three years earlier. I spoke with her friend on the phone outside near the soccer field, while Sarah was at practice. The friend insisted that orthopedists will not diagnose this syndrome and suggested I call an anesthesiologist myself, without a referral. Apparently, this condition is "taboo" in the medical field.

My brother, an attorney, called. "Hey Deb, this condition is tricky. I've had two clients with CRPS go to litigation. Many docs don't believe CRPS is a real condition. They claim they only see this condition in the courtroom. Besides, orthopedists only want to deal with the broken bones and not the 'trash' cases like CRPS." Then he insisted, "You've got a family depending on you," as though I was clueless.

I was already deeply aware of my responsibilities. I was so deeply aware that it hurt. It hurts when you're unable to care for the ones you love. I continued to navigate my way through the medical community to get answers and to get better.

CHAPTER 2

Sand in the Hourglass

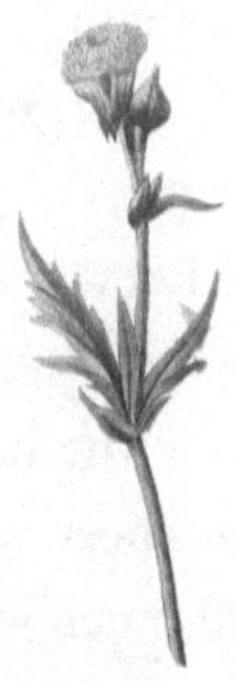

CARING EYES FOLLOWED ME as I was being wheeled away on a hospital gurney. "We love you!" my parents and John encouraged.

"I love you too!" I responded, trying to hide my fears. Tears ran down my cheeks as I rode farther down the long, cold hallway, watching them disappear. Thoughts of the needle entering my throat, injecting anesthetic meds into my cervical spine, filled my head with more horror than you can imagine. Paralysis was a risk I was willing to take to end or weaken the pain.

"How's your hand, Mrs. Kelly?" the anesthesiologist and his partner energetically visited my bedside after the injection, hoping to see progress. "Is the pain reduced? Do you have any movement?" they inquired. I felt like a science project.

"Don't *ever* touch my hand!" I screamed at the nurse who moved my arm. Nerve block number one was clearly unsuccessful.

"We'll try more nerve blocks for you, but we can only do a few. Come back in two days to get the next one. In the meantime, whatever you do, don't read about CRPS on the internet!" they jointly warned.

But they were too late, I had already read everything. After four more nerve blocks, the pain was reduced but not absent. Besides the nerve blocks, I was given a prescription for two medications: a steroid and a pack of gabapentin (also known as Neurontin). At the time, I knew gabapentin was a drug used to treat seizures and nerve pain. I was unaware it was also used to treat nerve pain caused by the herpes virus or shingles, as written on the information sheet with my prescription. This information eluded me until much later.

I was grateful for these interventions because acupuncture and occupational therapy had proven to be torture. But only about ten minutes into the anesthesiologist appointment, I was diagnosed with CRPS. It was a 180-degree turnaround from the orthopedist's office. The nerve blocks allowed for much more activity with my dominant hand. I could brush Sarah's hair into a ponytail and hold a book with both hands to read to her. I signed Evan's school papers and could turn the ignition key to start my car, which meant I was even able to help out by driving Sarah's carpool to school. I could open the mailbox, hold our dog Fluffy, zip up a sweatshirt, and gently embrace my husband. I shaved my legs with my right hand! I put on a watch and a bracelet by myself! The watch was an hour behind, since I'd missed daylight saving time. I had missed so many things over a three-month period.

I was also able to participate in some end-of-school activities, where I saw lots of people I'd missed. They were so concerned, asking how I was doing, and telling me they'd been praying for me. One of my favorite teachers told me two other teachers were crying and telling her how they had never seen me so down. They were used to seeing me often, smiling and in control amid the elementary school hallways. I had been absent until one day in the school's workroom, when a special teacher made the mistake of asking me how I was doing. I stopped in my tracks, weeping, and explained how I didn't know if this pain would ever go away. I told her that I'd been in the deepest darkest place I'd ever experienced, like being trapped in a well and wanting a way out. I thanked her for the prayers.

Research on CRPS consistently reported a better chance of remission or reduction in pain with treatment within six months of the initial injury. Already three months had passed, and I only had three months left to make a full recovery. Therapy became my focus for the summer. Mentally, there was a race with the calendar. I tried shielding the kids from as much as possible. They knew that Mom had a broken bone, but they didn't know the depth of my burning pain. They saw me in bed, with the curtains drawn, in pajamas all day, wearing my glasses instead of contacts, and overall looking horrendous day in and day out. I even wrote in my journal how *this may be misdiagnosed as chronic fatigue.* It seemed all I did was sleep and attend therapy. John was between jobs and thought he was going to have a fun-filled summer with the family. Instead, he was forced to take over, acting as both Mom and Dad, uncomfortably filling my shoes. Patrick, Evan, and

Sarah didn't know what to make of this sudden command change. John was driving all three kids around. Things were definitely out of order in our household.

I had arranged for Sarah's babysitter to come to our house to teach swim lessons to Sarah and her friend. The friend's mother was very confused when John answered the door.

"Where is Deborah?" she asked John.

"I'm sorry, but she's in bed asleep again," John honestly answered.

My bed was only ten feet away from the pool, but in the two-week period of swimming lessons, I'd only watched a lesson and visited with the other mom once.

"Is Mom dying?" Patrick asked John and me with a concerned look on his face. He was sitting in the living room and watching TV. I was in my robe, walking to the kitchen in the middle of the day after yet another nap. John had just walked in from picking Evan up at his friend's house. I suppose being the oldest, he was more aware of the changes at home.

"No, Mom isn't dying, Patrick," John soothed. "Her doctors are helping her, and she needs to rest often," he quickly responded.

"I'm just very tired, sweetheart, and I have to go to therapy to help my hand." I wasn't attuned to lying to my children, but we didn't know what was happening or what was going to happen. No one could tell us the cause of my condition. Making my children scared did not seem productive. If anything, his question motivated me to be discreet and not let them hear me complain. I tried not to show them how fearful I was. I often thought part of God's plan included John having a break between jobs, so he could be home. Both of our moms kept telling John that I must be depressed. But I didn't feel depressed—I felt tired. I felt really, really, really, really tired, like I had never felt before. I also felt an overwhelming desire to save myself and all the other people with CRPS.

My hand therapist and I established a pretty good rapport, until I spoke with one of his other patients who was sitting next to me one day. It was a young guy in his early twenties. I've always had the gift of gab, so striking up a conversation wasn't out of the ordinary. I asked him about his injury, and he asked me about mine. He then said he had asked the therapist if he would get the same disease I had. According to this young man, the therapist assured him he wouldn't get CRPS because it was only something "high-strung" people get, and he was very "chill." The therapist lost total credibility in my eyes. Not to mention, he admitted having a "special relationship" with several doctors in the area to keep his business flourishing.

If the actual therapy was making a difference, I would've continued to see him, but it simply wasn't. He confessed to only treating one other CRPS patient, and he often made fun of her with a story about her wig falling off during treatment. I asked the anesthesiologist for a therapist suggestion. He recommended the lady in the office next to him, so I went for a few visits. She was a loony tune who was scattered and micromanaging the office. She often sat me in a corner, doing odd hand exercises. The one cool thing she offered was mirror therapy, but I needed something better than what she was offering.

The sand in the hourglass was falling rapidly as that six-month deadline quickly approached. The only doctor I trusted was our family friend back in Louisiana. He suggested I find a certified hand therapist (CHT). At last, I found Helen, my new therapist, nearby. Her office was a breath of fresh air, with sunshine streaming in through the windows, framed groupings of butterflies on the wall, and rehab equipment neatly lying about.

Helen knew what she was doing. She was very professional and confident in her practice. She was always on time and got straight to business. On our first visit, Helen performed a specific evaluation measuring the range of motion of all the joints in both my hands. She gave me homework of specific exercises and stretches. She said stoplights were a great time to stretch my hand when in the car. She told me about the "scrub and carry" method, developed by H. Kirk Watson and Lois Carlson specifically for patients with CRPS.

Helen explained the "scrubbing" as using a scrub brush, kitchen sponge, or rag and getting down on your hands and knees to scrub in a back-and-forth motion. The "carry" portion of the method simply involved carrying heavy items. The "scrub and carry" method promoted movement and compression of an affected joint. It aimed to help patients regain function using weight-bearing and nerve stimulation. I was amazed this simple technique could be taught to CRPS patients and be done for *free*! John decided to invest ten dollars in a piece of plywood and a scrub brush for me to therapeutically scrub at home. I was so motivated to help those cases I'd read about, where people were suffering greatly but were without resources. The "scrub and carry" method was a technique for them!

Attending therapy three times a week was like going to work. I anxiously awaited each joint measurement that Helen took at the start of each session. I told John that therapy was like walking up a mountain backward because my progress was unclear. I wondered if more nerve blocks would do any good. There were days when I was so tired and dizzy that I wanted to crawl back in bed, but I pushed forward to make my appointments or take the kids somewhere. Time wasn't on my side. More than anything, I wanted my hand back, pain-free and fully functioning. The medications combined with the nerve blocks made therapy tolerable. Before those interventions, I had even thought about amputation when I drove by a prosthesis shop. The ongoing pain kept my mind wondering when, and if, I would recover.

"Hi Deborah, how are you doing? Ever since I read your email, I've been wanting to tell you about Allison," said my neighbor Elena, whom I ran into at an end-of-the-school-year awards ceremony.

"I'm doing okay. I've started therapy," I explained. "What did you want to tell me about Allison?" I asked. Allison was Elena's daughter who was in the same grade as Patrick.

"Two years ago, Allison had a broken bone in her foot. After going to three different doctors, she received the correct diagnosis of CRPS. Then, after five months of physical therapy, she was back to normal. We know exactly what you are going through."

Elena was the only person who told me, "I know you will get full functioning back, since you've come this far already." She will never know how much her words changed my outlook and filled me with hope. I tucked her encouragement under my cap and was determined to reach one hundred percent recovery.

I was geared to master any new therapy tools that Helen would offer, but after five weeks, she announced my therapy prescription was almost expired. How could that be? I felt that my right hand was nowhere near close to normal. Every morning as I woke up and lay in bed, I would think, *Is my hand better today?* Then I would try to move it, but it was still stuck. I had to bounce my fingers and warm them up to gain movement . . . every morning, every day. Helen said she didn't see any outstanding signs of CRPS. However, she didn't see my hand turn blue when I was in a cold building. She only asked about my pain level prior to therapy and never when the pain escalated during a session or movement.

Helen was only focused on what she could see and not what I was feeling. She thought I could continue "scrub and carry" at home and resume yoga. I argued that I didn't think I could do a downward dog pose. The thought of placing my full body weight on my right wrist was frightening. Helen asked if I had tried. I told her that I couldn't even push a grocery cart straight! I had to use my elbows when the cart was getting heavy or to round the corners of the aisles. I couldn't open a bottle of water or a jar. She had me lean on the table and do standing push-ups. I was favoring my left hand and cried in sheer frustration and pain. I was so angry, frustrated, and scared. I felt she was happy to get rid of me. She had already told me she didn't want to hear about my children or anything else I had to say, and that her next patient was one of her favorites.

I was on the brink of a nervous breakdown. I got in my car but couldn't drive home. I drove to the park behind our house. I parked the car and screamed as loudly as I could within the confines of the car's windows. Then I feared a man walking nearby would hear me. I sat there alone, unsure of whom to turn to next. I felt disconnected, looking up at the sunshine for warmth and at the lake to soothe me as only nature can do. I watched people playing with their children at the park, chasing the ducks and jogging along the path. I couldn't stay there; I had to get myself together before returning home. I couldn't look my husband in the eye. I knew he was tired of listening to me, so I focused on the kids' needs instead of my desperation. I was tired of it all too. That evening, Helen called me at home and apologized for not being able to tell me how my hand would progress. When I tucked Sarah into bed, she prayed, "God, please make my mom's hand feel better and make her happy again and more comfortable." Her prayer was a reminder that I wasn't alone and had to continue to trust this pain was for a greater purpose.

On my last occupational hand therapy session, Helen coached me to continue doing the stretches, strengthening exercises, and "scrubbing" at home. She mentioned that some CRPS patients attend therapy for years. But Elena had just shared that Allison was in therapy for five months. Why was I only given six weeks of therapy? I wanted to be empowered, so I asked her to keep working with me and show me more exercises. I called the second orthopedist's office and asked for a new therapy prescription. His office faxed the orders over to Helen's office without even asking to see me for a visit.

I was beginning to understand the rarity of my situation, in that health professionals were inconsistent and ill-educated about this problem. My anesthesiologist said he only saw about two cases a year and knew nothing about the "scrub and carry" technique. I told him he needed to know about it so he could help with the few cases he saw each year. He shared a story about someone in the UK who didn't have her first nerve block until two years after CRPS set in, which didn't do her much good. (I had read this condition needs immediate attention.) The doctor didn't think more nerve blocks would help me, and he didn't prescribe any more medication. I relied on what I'd learned in therapy. I did go back to see Helen several weeks later, but my insurance didn't cover the thirty-minute appointment, and the payment was several hundred dollars. That's the last time I saw Helen.

Outside of therapy, life kept going. John was preparing for the beginning of a start-up company in the oil and gas industry. He'd met with a financial advisor who suggested increasing the life insurance policy on me so he could start the business. That night I helped Sarah study for her science test. We joked that, in my absence, he would have to hire a nanny, a tutor, and upgrade Amber to a full-time chef. I was still unable to fulfill all my roles. John had taken over my unfinished household chores, but it was very difficult for me to let go. I wanted to be back from the black hole of CRPS. But at the end of the summer, I was able to bring Evan to camp about forty-five minutes away!

"Ev, it was so awesome to watch your fifth- and sixth-grade team win the championship game yesterday! I was so proud of you this season as you built trust with your teammates, and you all worked hard to improve and play as a unit," I exclaimed, thinking I was so glad I didn't miss the last game.

"We are ballers, Ma. High-five!" Evan replied, as I drove.

"Not today, Ev, my wrist really hurts. But don't you worry, I'll be able to dribble a basketball and score on you in no time," I joked.

"That'll never happen! You can't even do a single push-up. And you have to use that weird knob to turn the steering wheel. When will you be able to drive without that knob?" he wondered, motioning to the knob attached to the steering wheel.

"I wish I could tell you. Some people with this condition go to therapy for years, and for others, it never gets better," I said, pondering if I'd said too much. "I've been inspired to write a book," I revealed.

He'd been reading the notes on my phone about what great players he and Patrick were becoming and then replied, "Your book will be a *New York Times* bestseller. I dare you to write it! You'll be famous," he challenged.

"We are all already famed in God's eyes, according to Francesca Battistelli's song 'He Knows My Name,'" I answered.

"Ooooh, good one! Are you almost finished making something with your board?" he asked, referring to my plywood board.

"Evan, the board is for my therapy. It's supposed to help my hand," I answered, surprised he was unaware. Clearly, my children were confused. They saw me "scrubbing" on my hands and knees for ten to fifteen minutes each time. The motion always lessened the pain and had remained beneficial for eighteen months.

Besides "scrubbing," I relied on over-the-counter pain medications because I didn't want to become addicted to the narcotic pain medications I was prescribed. I had to drive and knew prescription pain meds did not mix well while driving with my kids in the car. Honestly, they didn't put a dent in the pain I felt anyway. Also, I didn't have a gabapentin prescription to mask the symptoms anymore. The anesthesiologist warned it wasn't a drug for long-term use and had a laundry list of side effects. Other symptoms came into the picture: low-grade fevers, fluctuating degrees of energy and pain, dizziness, days I couldn't get out of bed, interrupted sleep, insomnia, and migraines. I had turned to friends for suggestions, because my time limit was nearing as the sand kept dropping.

I went to a craniosacral therapist who told me I was healed after the second session, but truly there was no improvement. Another friend suggested her naturopath, Erin. Our many appointments were done over the phone, and she charged by the minute, so it wasn't cheap. She used something called Quantum Technique codes, which were a series of letters I was instructed to repeat out loud several times a day. As crazy as it sounds, I tried it. In the end, this did nothing for me. She also used charts to muscle-test various foods and toxins.

Muscle testing, also known as applied kinesiology, is a way of using muscles to find out what foods, supplements, and environmental factors are weakening or strengthening the body. Usually, this is done in person and used mostly by chiropractors, therapists, and holistic and functional medicine practitioners. In person, they would put an object near your body, then move your arm or leg in a certain position and apply pressure in an attempt to move your limb. Your muscle would remain strong, and your limb would be unable to be manipulated by the doctor or practitioner if the tested item strengthened the body. But if the tested item was a problem for you, your muscle would weaken, and your limb would easily be pushed down. Since our visits were on the phone, Erin used her limb on my behalf to do the testing remotely.

Through her testing, Erin encouraged me to cut out multiple foods, such as wheat products, corn products, refined sugar, oils, and dairy, and to change my household products with neurotoxic side effects, such as my popular laundry detergent and household cleaning supplies. This was all new to me, and I struggled with what I could eat. I read multiple books about CRPS, where the authors mostly wrote about ways to deal with the pain. I searched for a book with answers to completely eliminate the pain but came up short. Nicole Hemmenway revealed in her book, *No, It Is Not In My Head*, that a healthy diet and drinking seaweed juice were key to her getting out of a wheelchair and running a half-marathon. Maybe changing my diet was the right answer. I immediately stopped eating the foods Erin listed. It took a while to get into a new rhythm with foods I could eat. I scoured the grocery store aisles, reading ingredient lists and being very careful about what I bought to put into my body. I used to grocery shop according to what we liked by taste and wanted to eat. I began grocery shopping for foods to rejuvenate my health.

Erin was the first therapist to suggest dietary changes, but she couldn't explain *why* they would help, other than that the foods caused inflammation. I didn't understand why these foods would suddenly now be causing inflammation, because I had eaten them for forty-two years without a problem. She once coached me to let go of the diagnosis and allow healing to take place. With a nursing background, however, I firmly believed a proper diagnosis was instrumental for finding a cure. Erin also pointed to the word "conceal" on one of her charts. This left me wondering if I had some unresolved repressed issues that I was concealing. I continued the supplements she suggested until another practitioner cautioned against them, saying one could be toxic and radioactive with the aluminum heavy metal. Research became an ongoing effort, and I was willing to try anything.

One CRPS article described solanine toxicity. I read that solanine is a chemical present in the nightshade class of foods and is believed to aggravate arthritis pain and inflammation. Popular foods in the nightshade family are believed to be white potatoes, tomatoes, eggplant, all peppers, any red spice, and the ashwagandha herb. When I googled more about nightshades, I came across a chiropractor named Dr. Levi Mabrey, who seemed to be quite knowledgeable about solanine toxicity. Thinking this may be an answer to my prayers, I emailed him for an appointment. At the time, however, he only lectured and saw professional athletes. He was located states away, but his nephew, Hugh, saw me in Austin. Hugh used the muscle testing format and gave me several new supplements to take home. He encouraged avoiding most of the same foods Erin suggested, including nightshades. I always thought those foods were healthy. I thought all vegetables were healthy to eat. They were grown in the ground, for goodness' sake. Was I mistaken, or could the nightshades be migraine triggers? I suppose I adopted a paleo style of eating. I was never a migraine sufferer until this period in my life, post the five nerve blocks.

One evening, we took the boys shopping for summer camp and out to dinner. I accidentally had bell peppers on my grass-fed beef patty, even though I had been avoiding them as a nightshade veggie. That night, I felt poorly. I went into my daughter's room to cry myself to sleep in peace. I didn't want to worry about what my husband thought. In our almost eighteen years of marriage, that had never happened. I was so tired of feeling poorly. I had assumed that because my hand was getting stronger, the CRPS was going to diminish. But what if it didn't? Even if my wrist gained movement, flexibility, and strength, there was no guarantee that the condition would subside. I contemplated, *Is this how my life will be from now on?*

My daughter was at camp, and her room, which was set apart from the upstairs bedrooms, had become my safe haven. It was above the three-car garage, had a sitting room with a trundle, study table, and bathroom. Her bed was up a few steps under the triangular roof line. It was cozy, quiet, and private. The sizzling pain rumbled through my entire body. I tossed uncomfortably for half the night, saying prayers before settling to rest.

The next morning, my hand was noticeably swollen like a claw. I had tremendous pain at the base of my skull and a low-grade temperature. The temp was the first noticeable symptom of something unexplainably wrong. Was my CRPS getting worse? My bra hurt when secured, and I could only tolerate loose clothing. My whole body was inflamed. My head felt like it was going to explode. *Am I dying?* I wondered. I knew I couldn't live this way, with this much pain. My hope was gone. I felt paralyzed. I wanted to crawl back in bed and hide from the world.

I refer to that night as "my darkest night"—when I became even more hypersensitive to everything I put in my mouth. But accidents happen, and along came migraine number two. I had eaten crab and guacamole over lettuce for lunch, since oil and salad dressings were a no-no. Then I went with John and Evan to look at guitars. Evan thought it was so cool how his camp counselor played the guitar. But within an hour, I was dizzy with extreme head pain. The loud music ricocheted in my head like a pinball machine. John and Evan went to a movie, but I went home and got in bed. I felt like someone had hit me in the back of the head with a baseball bat as hard as they could. My head actually hurt to lie against the pillow, but the stillness felt better than motion. Drapes closed, lights off, and quiet was a necessity. Fortunately, I fell asleep, then woke up, walked to the refrigerator, and read there were jalapeño peppers in the guacamole.

A few days later came migraine number three. John and I had massages to celebrate our anniversary. The therapist said the entire right side of my body was holding much of my tension. Maybe she worked my body too hard. I ended up in bed the rest of the day, plagued with a headache and dizziness. The dizziness reminded me of my grandmother's vertigo. She used to complain when my cousins and I would spin around in her chairs. My poor ninety-four-year-old grandma was in a nursing home then with Alzheimer's disease. I wondered if the vertigo was a symptom of neurotoxicity that preluded Alzheimer's. Lying still in bed was all I could do. I watched countless episodes of *Say Yes to the Dress* and *Fixer Upper.* The volume remained very low because even loud noises hurt. I had hoped to sleep it off and feel better the next day because Sarah was returning home from her week away at camp and was always full of energy. This wasn't how I hoped to spend the day. I needed to go to the grocery store, but the jarring car ride would have been unbearable.

On our anniversary, August 6, 2012, I felt much better. I noticed a pattern following a migraine, day in bed, or nightshade episode. It took two days to recover. I had good days and bad; no wonder my family and friends thought I was crazy. By the time migraine number four of the summer presented itself, John had taken the kids to lunch, as my head hurt to walk or be upright. I hoped that if I rested for two days, I'd be better the following day. I did have some good days, but it was hard to pace myself on those days because I had energy and always seemed behind on what needed to be done. I had to let a lot of things go by the wayside.

I pampered my body, getting pedicures with Sarah from a place using vegan supplies. I couldn't tolerate the noxious smells at regular nail salons. I nourished my soul, listening to our local Christian radio station, KSBJ. I connected with the song "Where I Belong" by the group Building 429. It became my personal theme song. I was lost, and no one from this world seemed to have answers for me. I needed spiritual superpowers to help me find my way home.

CHAPTER 3

What Now?

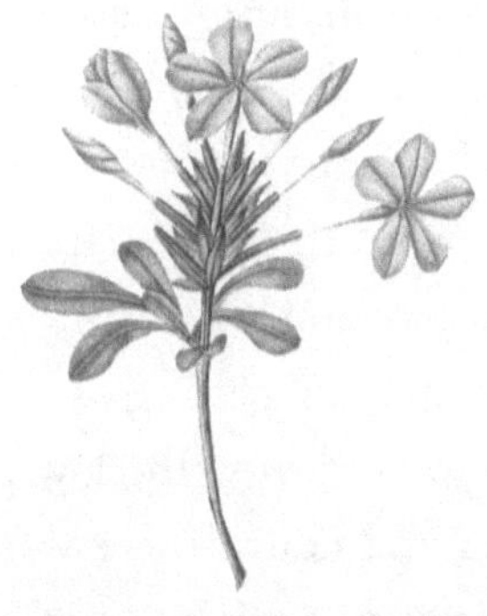

My CRPS six-month time frame came and went. Someone mentioned I should be thankful that I didn't have brain lesions like her friend, Terri, from the beauty shop. Well, guess what? I wasn't thankful. I didn't feel more fortunate than Terri because I did not feel normal. I was petrified of living with chronic pain for the rest of my life. Every doctor or therapist said something different, and there was no guarantee it was ever going to go away. I had spoken with people who completely healed over months or years, in addition to others who still continued to live with CRPS pain and symptoms long-term.

Every day was different. My symptoms varied in number and intensity. I couldn't rely on making plans. I was in survival mode and preserving energy for my family. When I woke up every morning, I didn't know if I would make it through that day. I didn't know if I would be able to get things done or if my body would require sleep for several more hours. I didn't know if I would be too dizzy to drive or in too much pain to think straight. It became common to accomplish only one or two of many errands. I always felt behind or had to simplify or leave things undone. A good day was having diminished pain in my head or hand and having an intact stamina. People would see me one day looking fine and then not understand why I couldn't get out of bed the following day or that afternoon. Believe me, this is more frustrating for the patients than for their friends and families.

After taking a shower and getting dressed, I would be totally exhausted and have to lie down. The low-grade fevers and ibuprofen popping persisted daily. There was no staying up late, or my body would retaliate with bouts of insomnia. I felt like a radioactive bomb about to go off at any time. A sign displayed in the drive-thru car wash—HIGH VOLTAGE, DANGER!—reminded me of my nervous system. My days were filled with thoughts of lessening the pain in any form or fashion. My defenses were up, as I was unaware what symptoms would appear at any given moment. My adrenaline was in full gear. After time passed, John shared with me that I had frequent mood changes. I didn't realize it then. My mood simply reflected how I felt on the inside—no one can feel your insides; they can only experience the outside. Modern medicine did what it could for me, then tossed me out to pasture. Once again, I turned to others for help.

One friend suggested I see her chiropractor. He offered me a blood test, the results of which indicated a list of foods to eat, a list of foods to avoid, and a list of foods to eat sparingly. He said usually wheat and corn pop up across the board on everyone's list of foods to avoid. He sounded just like dog food commercials promoting no corn or wheat in their products. He mentioned taking the test annually because toxicities build up over time and cause inflammation. There was that word again, *inflammation.* I wove those test results into my diet, and Amber cooked using my "good food" list, but it only narrowed further what I could eat and added to my stress.

"Deborah, what about everything in moderation? Now, you can hardly eat anything!" John balked. He was struggling with my dietary restrictions.

"I'm trying anything I can to heal and get rid of this pain. Besides, some of the foods make me hurt worse!" I retorted.

"Remember when we talked about exploring new restaurants in the city when I would be off work this summer? That's something I thought we would be able to do together," he expressed.

"I'm trying to get back to normal," I pled.

Frannie, John's mom, tried to help. She told us about her neighbor who went to Vero Beach, Florida, seeking treatment for CRPS. Her neighbor saw Dr. Hooshmand and was placed on a special diet. This doctor encouraged eating the four Fs: fresh fruit, fresh vegetables (if cooked, only in olive oil), fish (baked or broiled without butter), and fowl (not fried). He also preached avoiding the five Cs: cookies, cake, chocolate, cocktails, and candy. Incorporating the four Fs and avoiding the five Cs had already been woven into my diet, minus my temptation for dark chocolate. When I called to inquire about an appointment, the receptionist explained the doctor was no longer treating CRPS patients because insurance wasn't accepting CRPS as a diagnosis. Another medical dead end, yet I was at the start of something different.

I didn't realize it at the time, but I was beginning to use food as medicine. Hippocrates, the famous Greek physician, is considered to be the father of modern medicine. He saved Athens from a plague epidemic and scientifically described his observations of many diseases in over seventy books. Hippocrates is credited with the quote: "Let food be thy medicine, and let medicine be thy food." Food does more than provide us with fuel. It holds the power to promote or worsen our health.

Later I learned about the emotional ties that we have with food revolving around our daily lives, traditions, and holidays. At this point in my journey, I was treading water but took the food-related suggestions seriously, even though it was difficult. I had to do something! I thought if I followed all the diet advice, I might actually heal. I frequented the farmers' market for grass-fed beef and eggs from pasture-raised chickens with access to eating grass, bugs, and worms. I had been instructed to stick with grass-fed beef, as a means of cutting out the grains eaten by cattle, because grains cause *inflammation*. Essentially, whatever the animal eats, you eat. Unfortunately, the one restaurant in our area serving grass-fed beef closed. Grass-fed beef was generally more expensive, and restaurants are in business to make money.

We took trips to our local seafood market for fresh fish and shrimp. Our favorites were grilling redfish, sauteing shrimp, and baking sea bass. Figuring out what I could and couldn't eat was trial and error. I tried some gluten-free pancakes, which were absolutely terrible, even with all the maple syrup in the world. It seemed most gluten-free foods substituted wheat with a corn product. Both wheat and corn were off the table for me, literally. It was shocking how many products found on the grocery store shelves included gluten and corn as fillers in their ingredients. I went to the local health market for specialty foods and to buy new supplements to try. They suggested I try an ionic foot bath for detoxification. The water in my foot baths would turn from crystal clear to black with green and burnt orange deposits. The workers proclaimed I must've felt horrible, because the color revealed more *inflammation* than they had ever seen. Soaking my feet in water felt nice, but my pain persisted.

Going out to eat was a challenge. It was a big day when I had lunch at a local deli chain. I ordered a side of chopped turkey and a fruit cup without pineapple because it was on my "bad food" list. Then, the host of additives, phosphates, and fillers in deli meat were unknown to me. For a crunch, I brought a handful of almonds along with my lunchtime supplements. Bringing my own food if we ate out or at someone's home became the norm. A few times, I tried ordering in restaurants, however, the list of items to remove was never completely communicated from me to the waiter and back to the kitchen. I'd always find red pepper seasoning, added oils, or something else in my food that could possibly trigger pain or a migraine.

Friends often acted uncomfortable when I brought my own food to restaurants. When people go to a restaurant, they want to eat for pleasure and not think about health benefits or detriments. My friend was about to order a fried chicken sandwich with fries but switched her order to a salad after seeing me remove my salad from my lunchbox. Another friend was married to a restaurant manager and explained that people aren't allowed to bring their own food because it wasn't up to food safety codes. That day, I ate at home before meeting our group. Later, I learned from my friend Shannon that under the Americans with Disabilities Act of 1990, one should be allowed to fully participate in society with public accommodations as medically necessary. When I say I've brought my food due to too many allergies, I usually don't have a problem.

It was a great night when Amber surprised me with savory garlic sauce topped buckwheat noodles for dinner at home. She also created a pumpkin and beet sauce with Italian seasoning to mimic a red sauce, since I couldn't eat tomatoes as a nightshade. She was becoming highly creative in the kitchen! One of the toughest parts of following my new diet was the lack of social eating. My parents and John didn't understand why I wouldn't eat bread. They didn't comprehend how it was affecting my nervous system. I wasn't exactly sure either. When you take bread out of an American diet, your food options become limited. When my family went out for pizza, I'd go to the grocery store. My food limits were inconveniently isolating me from family and friends further. My lunchtime sandwich became a thing of my past.

One Saturday night, we had a business dinner meeting with John's coworkers at an upscale steak restaurant. Before we arrived, he asked, "What will you order? Spinach?" He wanted this dinner to run smoothly.

I was upset by his question, thinking spinach without a salad dressing would taste horrible. I wasn't a rabbit. My taste buds were unaltered. He seemed to have forgotten it was my nervous system and hand I was trying to correct.

"I previewed the menu, and the steaks aren't grass-fed, so a salad may be all I can eat. I can't have a salad dressing because their dressings have oil and vinegar. I'll have to ask the waiter about the salad toppings. I don't know what they put in their soups, and they don't have anything else from my safe edible list."

I ended up eating a plate of spinach topped with pears and pecans without dressing, while the rest of the table devoured their juicy steaks, warm and buttered homemade dinner rolls and all the sides, washed down by fine wines. But it was the conversations revolving around the food that bothered me the most.

"What's today's special? How do you like your steak cooked? May I suggest this such-and-such wine? What are you going to order? Such-and-such restaurant in Paris served the finest steak that I've ever had. These scalloped potatoes are better than my grandma's version. Next time, we should go to this such-and-such restaurant on the west side of town." All non-pertaining to me. All of it. It was torture and a reminder I wasn't normal.

Another time, we went to a Brazilian steakhouse for a friend's birthday. This was the type of restaurant where the waiters brought several types of meat to the table until you gave them a signal to stop. Everyone had a card at their place setting with a green "Go" side and a red "Stop" side. I kept my card on the red side. Of course, I had eaten at home before the celebration. For some reason, our waiters ignored my red card. It was hard enough not to participate in the meal, but to have to constantly tell the waiters I didn't want the meat was simply a giant nuisance. On the other hand, our kids had a wonderful time and were so happy to finally go out to dinner.

A few times, friends would accompany us to a seafood restaurant where I could order baked fish without butter and steamed vegetables. Soon, however, they wanted to go elsewhere, or I wasn't feeling well enough to join them, so our outings quickly fizzled. Dates with John were going to the movies with my earplugs and sunglasses (to dampen the loud narrative and bright screen) and a bag of grapes to snack on since they were quiet to chew.

Other foods that were heavenly enticing were the pastries brought by the grandmothers, Millie and Frannie. Every time they visited, they brought French bite-sized petit fours cakes and large doberge multi-layered cakes from their favorite bakeries in Louisiana. They visited often to celebrate birthdays and holidays and to watch the kids play sports. It seemed like we had cakes on hand every other month. They could've potentially been the best things that I had ever eaten, but I had to repeatedly keep my willpower up time and time again.

"I stopped at the bakery on the way. The cake needs to be refrigerated," they'd say. "But you can keep the little petit fours out on the counter for the kids."

"Sure, I can do that," I politely responded. Then I did as requested, sorting the temptation into my home for them to enjoy. But instead of eating the little bits of deliciousness, I inhaled the familiar smell of buttercream icing mixed with almond and vanilla flavoring until my heart was content.

Things were about to change at home. John had been diligent, getting detail after detail settled prior to opening the doors of his new start-up company. On a slow walk with my friend, Natalie, I confided, "I don't know how I'll keep up with the demands of the kids' upcoming school schedule. John is going back to work. I don't have enough energy to do everything."

Natalie was (and still is) a firecracker and a problem solver. We've raised our kids together, lived near one another, and attended church together. She's petite in stature with a huge sense of humor and zest for learning. She's always up on current events as she scours the news and reads constantly for pleasure and knowledge. For me, she's been a faithful friend who called often just to check on me and never treated me differently. Once I told her my concerns, she went into action.

First, she contacted our mutual friend, Sabrina, and planned a visit for the three of us at her home. Sabrina was a close friend, yet had been distancing herself for quite some time, especially since my accident. While the three of us were visiting at Natalie's home, Sabrina never asked how I was doing and mainly spoke about her family and job. I was under the impression that she wasn't interested in maintaining our relationship as I had become high-maintenance. My hand was burning like crazy that day, and I was filled with emotions of sadness, frustration, and abandonment, but I looked perfectly normal. CRPS was a hard concept to explain and to grasp. Nevertheless, the visit prompted a reality check as friends began drifting away.

Second, Natalie offered to speak with her uncle, a neurologist, about my case. Her uncle connected me with another neurologist whose office was located in the Houston Medical Center, an hour away. John and I met the neurologist in the lobby of his clinic. I suppose he was fitting me into his schedule.

Within seconds of viewing my right hand, he proclaimed, "Yes, I can tell you have CRPS in your right hand. I can see it plainly! What I can do is surgically install a neurostimulator implant, which we'll use to treat chronic pain. The implant will positively give you a fifty percent increase in your hand's mobility."

He then proceeded to explain in detail the surgical procedure, but red flags were surfacing in my mind! *Why was he so quick with a diagnosis, just like the anesthesiologist, when the orthopedist shied away from one? Why was he more interested in explaining the surgical procedure, and why didn't he listen to any of my symptoms?* I wondered. The risk versus reward was unclear.

Following the hour's drive back home, the phone rang. "I'm returning a call to a Deborah Kelly. I'm with the RSD Hope Foundation."

"Yes sir, thank you for calling me back. I've had five nerve blocks, and I just met with a neurologist about a neurostimulator implant," I stated to the foundation's representative.

"Oh no! Whatever you do, avoid neurostimulators and infusion pumps at all costs, and run the other way if anyone else offers you one! I've seen multiple people mutilated from these procedures, which are big moneymakers for doctors," he emphatically warned. He had suffered with RSD for twenty-six years and was currently recovering from a left leg amputation.

I found out that the side effects from the procedure included risk of neurologic injury, allergic reaction to the device, spinal puncture, and pain itself. It didn't seem like a very smart idea to treat chronic pain with something able to induce pain and injury. Assuming the call was a blessing, I refused the neurostimulator.

Third, Natalie gave me a week pass to her female-only gym. She wanted me to try their infrared sauna, because it promised to penetrate the tissues deeper than a regular sauna and draw out toxins from the body. The literature on the infrared sauna was impressive. I read how the infrared sauna helped with chronic fatigue because it released metal toxicity. It was easy! There were three saunas in a backroom located near the showers. All I had to do was sit in the hot wooden box, wrapped in a towel, and sweat while reading magazines provided by the gym. One article I read reported that fifty-two percent of people found it easier to do their taxes than to eat healthily. I wondered to myself if that were sadly true.

The next morning, I was feeling hopeless until I was on the way to the hospital to responsibly visit Sabrina. She had a pulmonary embolism from her birth control and migraine medications, yet her prognosis and her spirits were upbeat. I was stretching my hand in the car at a stoplight as I usually did, then suddenly my hand bent forward! I couldn't believe my eyes. I didn't know if it would ever happen. I called John right away with the good news. Natalie was also visiting Sabrina, so I showed her the movement when I saw her at the hospital. She asked what I thought contributed to the bending. I guessed the supplements, diet change, scrubbing therapy, and the infrared sauna treatment I'd had the day before.

I joined the gym just to use the sauna. I went two to three times a week. It gave me *energy*! After a few sessions, I noticed that I could push a grocery cart evenly, with both hands, and not rely on my elbows to round the corners. You should have seen the smile on my face! I longed to be able to take part in the gym's exercise classes, but I settled for the relief from their sauna.

I began watching *Today with Kathie Lee and Hoda* as I spent much time at home alone. One of the show's guests shared her confusion as to why she got cancer since she had a healthy life-style. I contemplated her inquiry long and hard. I had thought about the same scenario when I heard about a fit jogger drop-ping dead of a heart attack. Everyone has toxins in their systems from foods, metals, pesticides, radiation, and medications. I hypothesized that possibly our metabolisms don't change. Per-haps our toxins simply build up in the body, causing disease or death. I was sold on the infrared sauna.

Fall was in the air as the kids were going back to school. Pat-rick was entering high school while Evan was entering junior high—both pivotal times at new schools. Fortunately, Sarah was entering third grade at the same elementary school that we held so dear. I wanted to be involved; I wanted to eagerly sign up on all those beginning-of-the-school-year lists. It was important for me to be present and feel the atmosphere where my children spent so much time, but I had to restrain myself to conserve my energy. I was grateful, however, for being able to take my boys to their orientations and touring the cold school halls.

A woman walking next to me at the high school advised, "You need to carry your purse with your other hand!"

"I sure will, thank you," I appreciated, noticing that my hand had turned purple. I thought I was finished with those CRPS symptoms of limb color and temperature changes. It reminded me of Raynaud's disease, which is also characterized by discol-orations of the hands and feet and feelings of numbness and cold. In nursing school, I diagnosed myself with this syndrome since my hands and feet were *always* cold. Friends and family members often gifted me with warm items like sweaters, blankets, and slippers. My purple hand seemed to be a sign of lacking progress; even so, I was thankful to be out of bed and participating in normal parenting life.

I tried keeping a normal routine. I was selected to be the co-room mom for Sarah's grade and was fortunate to work side by side with wonderful women. I was in the workroom at the elementary school on copy duty, but after forty-five minutes, I suddenly had the onset of a massive headache and weakness. I'd planned to go to the grocery store on the way home because our kitchen pantry and refrigerator needed refilling. But all I could do was head home to lie down, leaving the school's copy job for someone else. I hosted a football locker sign decoration event for Evan's grade with more fantastic moms, yet John had to deliver the signs when they were due because I was stuck in bed again. Another day, Patrick and his friend were working on their biology project. They needed to collect over one hundred bugs and leaves and weren't allowed to have parental assistance. I hadn't planned on helping them, but I wanted to know what supplies were needed and to make sure that they remained on task. I had no idea what they were doing, however, while I was aching in bed. Much to their credit, the boys did a terrific job! I was the one with the problem. I had to let go.

Although I was hardly volunteering at the schools, I had previous commitments to complete. At the end of the last school year, I had agreed to chair the junior high community project, as I had expected to be completely healthy by that time. The project was a food drive for the local women's shelter. It was an honor to collaborate in the fight against domestic violence. I asked God for assistance because I didn't want to fail on such an important job. Luckily, there were two Girl Scouts who attended the junior high and needed to fulfill hours for a service program. The Girl Scouts, along with their mothers, were the answer to my prayer and the boost I needed to make the project a success.

In between the morning and afternoon volunteer sessions, I collapsed at home, taking advantage of my downtime for rest, eating, and scrubbing hand therapy. It was so worth it. We filled a moving truck with food donations and proudly collected over $2,000 in monetary donations. Being around so many "normal" people made me realize I really had a long way to go. Overwhelmed with hopelessness, I was tired of living like I was on a rollercoaster. Without an end in sight, I often spoke with God multiple times a day, seeking His direction.

The donation collection week was wrapping up, and soon I'd be left without a distraction. I was in the junior high conference room, where I had found I had a few quiet minutes to myself. I asked, "God, when will I be normal again? When will this pain subside? I need you—I need help! I don't know where to turn. Can you give me a sign of hope? I need something to help keep me moving forward."

Hours later, I found a shiny penny on the floor. The imprinted phrase "IN GOD WE TRUST" loomed to my attention. That phrase on the coin was undoubtedly poignant. *I had to trust His plan.* I couldn't see any purpose to my pain, but I knew that God has a better view than we do. Proverbs 3:5–6 came into focus: "Trust in the Lord with all your heart, on your own intelligence rely not; in all your ways be mindful of him, and he will make straight your paths."

From that point onward, I found pennies everywhere, often during my worst moments. For some reason, I found pennies on the cement nearly every time I exited my car at the gas station and at the grocery store. I anxiously looked for them as they meant more to me than a single cent. They were reminders from above to trust that one day everything would be alright. My family shared the joy when they found the pennies too.

Daily life carried on with or without me. Fluffy was my faithful companion, always by my side. She especially kept me company, lying next to me in bed if it was a bedridden day. Petting her soft fur was therapy for my hand, and she loved the attention. Carpools were a lifesaver for the kids' after-school practices and lessons. I'm forever grateful for the mothers who carpooled with us and often took my turn.

Sometimes, I enjoyed visiting with the other parents, but other times, I just felt rotten. At one of Sarah's soccer practices, I was aching from head to toe. It was one of those days where I *had* to keep going, even though all the unseen "HIGH VOLTAGE, DANGER!" indicators in my painful body were blaring as loudly as they could. Ideally, I would've been at home in bed under the covers. It was a warm, cloudy day, and the usual crowd of parents had lined their chairs along the grassy soccer field. I simply couldn't tolerate any stimulation. I knew I had to sit alone, far away from the group, just to get through the practice without falling apart. I kept telling myself, *Just be still for one hour, and then you can go home.* Too vulnerable with pain, I feared engaging in eye contact and conversation with the other caring parents. I didn't think anyone would understand, and knowing I was on the brink of tears, I avoided them. The same thing happened at one of Evan's basketball games. I had arrived at the gym when the game began and sat at the very top of the bleachers with my back to the wall. I was seated far away from the other parents—away from interference. *Just be still for one hour, and then you can go home,* I thought.

A few weeks later, there was a significant difference. "Deborah, I'm going to have to leave the soccer tournament for a few hours, so can you please watch out for Megan while I'm gone?" asked Megan's mom.

"Sure, I'll be happy to. I'll be here all day," I assured her.

"I see you brought a salad, apple, almonds, dates, and carrots for lunch. Do you always eat this healthy?" another mom asked.

"I sure do. I'm using food as medicine to heal pain and fatigue," I answered.

"You know, in South America, the grocery stores mainly have fresh foods and not prepackaged foods like the U.S. grocery stores," two of the moms compared.

"The U.S. makes up ten percent of the world's population yet takes forty percent of the world's pharmaceuticals," the coach included.

I wasn't the only one interested in eating well and being healthy. Everywhere I turned, people were in severe pain, had high blood pressure and high cholesterol, suffered from anxiety and depression, and had other assorted issues. I was beginning to think eating healthily *could* be the best form of disease prevention and reversal, and I wasn't the only one noticing. That day, I made it through a whole day at Sarah's soccer tournament. It was so exciting because her team made it to the finals and won their age bracket.

In preparation for attending a special event, I'd stay purposefully home to save my energy. At one of those events, a football game, Evan was three for three in catching football passes. He even scored a touchdown after diving for one of those passes. Evan's teammates piled on him in excitement when he returned to the sidelines. He was on top of the world, and I was so glad to be there to witness it. It was also fun to participate in Patrick's first high school homecoming experience and see him and his friends dressed up and going out as a group with their dates. I was set apart from my family in so many ways, so I showed up when I was able to bridge the gaps.

However, even if I was physically present, there were times I wasn't mentally present. I was so exhausted sitting in the stands at Patrick's track meets several times that I wanted to stretch out on the bleachers and fall fast asleep. I actually did fall asleep when I brought Sarah and two friends to a local play of *The Little Mermaid*. When I awoke with a headache, the music, clapping, and crowd were just overstimulating. I made the girls follow me out of the theater quickly so I could get home immediately. I became more sensitive to noise, lights, smells, and chemicals and began having dizzy spells. Once, a natural shampoo from the grocery store threw me into slow motion with a monster headache. Another time, I had a sleepless night with a headache after a haircut. I wondered if the cause of my affliction was something I ate or perhaps the hairspray my hairdresser used, since she normally didn't use it. The following day, I took Evan for a haircut with the same person. When I asked her about the hairspray, she said she had other clients who also got headaches from the same product.

What was happening to me? I didn't understand, and fearfulness was mounting as several other symptoms gained in stride. My heart palpitations had grown in intensity. They came in the morning with racing speed, just as I opened my eyes. I would be lying still in bed, without exertion, and my heart would be thumping. Palpitations often came roaring in the night, keeping me awake for hours. Ear pain, numbness, and tingling sensations in my legs also occurred, coming and going each day. I worried that the CRPS was spreading to my legs and would leave me wheelchair dependent. My toes would become stiff, and the awful numbness and tingling sensations would radiate from my trunk downward to the tops of my feet. I questioned if my legs were going to turn purple like my hand often did, and in the mornings, I'd hesitantly lift the bedding just to check.

Sometimes, it felt as if an elephant were sitting on my big toe. I noticed that my leg pain seemed related to my activity level. If I was too active for a few days in a row, my body fought back. There were days when driving—simply pressing the car's accelerator or brakes—was a painful task. Then I'd have that rare, glorious day where I was able to drive an hour away to the Houston Ballet Nutcracker Market, a shopping extravaganza. I blamed all my odd issues on my CRPS, and I was still unsure of my future. In hindsight, I can now acknowledge several God winks (whispers of grace) that surfaced during that time. Natalie helped me find the infrared sauna, the Girl Scouts helped me with the fundraiser, I had begun finding pennies from heaven, and I'm still grateful for the warning about the neurostimulator.

Read for a Better Life

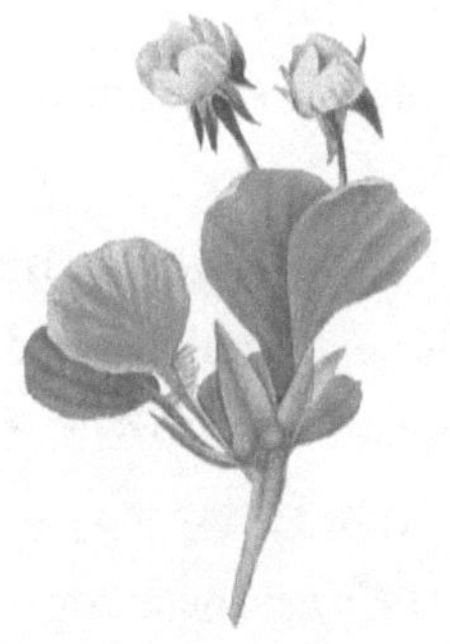

WHEN THE SYMPTOMS CULMINATED and I landed in bed, John stepped up. He took my place teaching Sarah's church class one Sunday because the other teacher was out of town. Later that afternoon, he found me still in my pajamas in bed, waking up from a deep sleep. He walked in with two strawberry-banana smoothies, one for each of us. I had no idea what time it was, but it wasn't dark outside yet. Fluffy rose from her own sweet spot by my leg and angled for some love from John as she licked his hands.

He appeased her and asked, "How do you feel?" He hated seeing me in such misery.

"Thank you for letting me sleep. I hope the church class went well. I'm not getting out of bed for dinner," I said. "I'll just have the smoothie."

"Okay, the class was fine. The same two little boys were throwing crayons at each other. You know, I would tell you to go see a doctor, but I know you won't go," he remarked.

I sat up against the pillows and argued, "Who would you like me to see? I've already been to doctors, and they can't help me!" He was acting as if I was being hardheaded. I thought finding a doctor well-versed in CRPS was like finding a needle in a haystack, and I had already sifted through that haystack.

"Well, you could go see the same chiropractor Libby went to for her leg pain," he rallied.

"Sure, why not? I'll make an appointment," I retorted. I was hopeful when this doc said all I needed was a few routine adjustments for sciatic pain. Unfortunately, the adjustments only brought temporary relief.

Then I went back to the anesthesiologist who had performed my five nerve blocks. He suggested an MRI, which could lead to steroid shots, but my neurological exam was clean. He couldn't explain the numbness, tingling, and pain, and said that CRPS doesn't spread from one limb to another. He was incorrect; I had already read everything on CRPS, and there were multiple cases of the condition spreading.

Next, it was time to visit orthopedist number two again. I reported the status of my right hand. The unpredictable levels of burning and pain had remained, yet I was able to open water bottles and jars and drive without the knob on my steering wheel. My hand had finally regained enough strength to turn the wheel. He announced the X-ray and CAT scan showed complete healing of the once-broken wrist bone. He asked if I was still doing anything to help my hand. I told him I was still doing the scrubbing therapy three times a day. I revealed my concerning heart palpitations, asking how to stop them.

"I have no idea," he answered. He suggested following up with my primary care physician.

I felt I only benefited from him when he wrote orders for the X-ray, CAT scan, and hand therapy. I wanted *more* from my doctors—more information, more knowledge, and more care in general for myself and other CRPS patients. I saw a nurse practitioner at my primary care physician's office for a well check. She asked who I was seeing for CRPS but didn't ask for any specifics. She was focused on getting through my physical exam and moving on to the next patient. On paper, all my lab work came back within the normal limits, but I was far from being normal. I was far from *where I belonged*, and my foundation was shaken.

Driving in the car with a friend, I shared my dilemma, "Everywhere I turn for help, there seems to be a barrier."

"Maybe you just need to accept your situation?" my friend concluded.

I had no reply as I glared out of the window, realizing my friend's advice was merely another barrier. I wanted to know *why* my body fell apart after I broke my wrist, and I wanted my life back. There were too many loose ends for me to throw in the towel.

I felt so alone in my journey and so misunderstood. But at an elementary school holiday party, a selfless male special needs teacher found me walking in the hallway, gathering up supplies.

"I want you to know I understand what you are going through," he softly spoke. "My wife passed a few months ago from CRPS."

"I'm so sorry, I had no idea," I said tenderly.

"Her body temperature was burning up all the time. I would turn the air conditioner on in her car before she could get inside. The CRPS caused her blood pressure to skyrocket, and she had to be on dialysis. When that didn't work anymore, she passed away," he lamented.

Tearfully, we exchanged a sympathy hug. We shared a moment of mutual compassion, despite his words leaving me terror-stricken. The kind of terror where you can hardly breathe. Then we were pulled into different classrooms, and we kept going, as mothers and teachers always do. Without answers, my future was dim. I *had* to fight to regain my life, or it would keep deteriorating.

At the same school party, two wonderful teachers approached me, assuring me they'd had similar pain issues and understood the mental and emotional impact. The caring duo gave me a referral, suggesting another teacher's cousin who was a chiropractor. Dr. Gram was certified in internal medicine and used muscle testing to get to the root of each problem. He had helped several of the teachers, so I made an appointment.

My mysterious internal inflammation endured. I hoped changing my diet was the answer—*the* cure. The diet changes helped but weren't enough. My favorite Christmas gifts that year were gluten-free cookbooks from a few friends. When I saw a friend over the holidays, she asked, "Are you okay? You are *so* thin. I have never seen you like this." I had lost over twenty pounds in six months but was *extremely* uncomfortable and miserable in my own skin. My journey wasn't about losing weight; it was about retrieving my health. My jeans were falling off my hips, so I went shopping for smaller sizes. Never did I dream I would have such a small pants size in my closet.

My food sensitivities had heightened. At a spontaneous New Year's Day dinner, I took a chance and drank half a glass of wine. I paid the consequences, however, with pain in my hand and leg and an inability to sleep. I thought a cup of chamomile tea at a movie theater concession stand would be safe, but mere moments after a few sips, my stomach ached. Tremendous head pressure developed after a bite of a gluten-free chocolate chip cookie. Dessert became unsweetened applesauce and non-dairy fruit smoothies. When our families brought those delectable French cakes over, I was tempted and thought a bite might be scrumptious. But I knew it wasn't worth jeopardizing my road to recovery. I tried making gluten-free pizza and muffins from tapioca, sorghum, and almond flour, yet my leg pains worsened. Sometimes after eating red meat, I felt like someone punched me in the stomach. I craved salt all the time, which I later learned was a sign of adrenal fatigue.

My dad, Jim, didn't understand gluten-free or grain-free foods and was concerned about my weight loss. Once a track star back in his day, he loved watching all the kids' sporting events. While visiting, he asked if I wanted a piece of cake, a sandwich, and a bowl of cereal—all in the same day. I gave him "the look" each time. He didn't know that gluten is a protein found in wheat and other grains. He utterly couldn't be bothered with such nonsense. He had always been tall and slim with long and narrow appendages. Yet as he aged, his belly grew larger with every bowlful of ice cream.

When he visited, he brought his own bag from the bakery, aside from the French cakes. His little white bakery bag would be filled with cookies, turnovers, lemon bites, and donuts for breakfast. His sweet tooth came from his grandfather, who owned a bakery. My dad kept a stash of candy in his car and on the side table next to his favorite living room chair. He was always on the go, living on his sugar high until the next meal. He had places to be and people to see, spreading his charismatic nature all around my Louisiana hometown.

My grandfather was a music professor, so Jim became a music store owner before his two other careers: a governmental agency president in south Louisiana for hurricane and flooding protection, and a contractor who built homes. He was always in charge, never bowing to authority, and he loved a good shortcut. Nutrition was far from interesting to him. He turned his nose up at most vegetables and anything green. He didn't understand my using food as medicine. He had always gone "through the back door" to his doctor friend when an injection or a prescription was necessary; no appointment needed.

John and I were the ones focused on what was (and what wasn't) going in my mouth. John wondered if the Catholic church had a gluten-free substitute for Holy Communion. I hadn't thought about the wheat in the host, but I did have a pattern of feeling rotten on Mondays following Sunday Mass. There is, in fact, a low-gluten or partially gluten-free substitute permitted in some areas. However, the smallest amount of gluten seemed to be a problem for me. From this point onward, I chose to receive a blessing instead of the wafer at Mass. It is difficult to break free from our rituals. I toiled with this decision, but ultimately, I focused on the God I know—a God whose love for us has no boundaries and no conditions. He is not a one-size-fits-all creator. He always has an open seat for us at His table. I focused on caring for the body God gave me and kept growing spiritually without the ritual.

Our school superintendent promoted the motto "Read for a Better Life." I was reading all I could to explore a way to better health. Dr. William Davis, author of *Wheat Belly*, encourages a wheat-free diet to prevent and reverse heart disease. He says that wheat affects every organ and system in our bodies, including the nervous system and brain. *Finally, a doctor who mentions wheat affecting us!*

Dr. Davis warns today's wheat products, including those used for religious ceremonies, don't contain the same grain our forefathers ground into their daily bread. He explains that modern wheat has been hybridized and genetically altered from "amber waves of grain" to an eighteen-inch-tall "dwarf" wheat, easily averaging a yield tenfold greater than furnished a century ago. He also believes the food industry's financial gains from the massive American wheat consumption led to "the 'need' for billions of dollars of drug treatments for diabetes, heart disease and all other health consequences of obesity." He says it's as if a powerful group in the mid-1950s mapped out "an evil plan to mass-produce high-yield, low-cost dwarf wheat, engineer the release of government-sanctioned advice to eat 'healthy whole grains' [and] lead the charge of corporate Big Food to sell hundreds of billions of dollars worth of processed wheat food products." Could it be the gains for certain men that marked mankind in poorer health?

What surprised me the most was reading that two slices of whole wheat bread could elevate blood sugar levels higher than drinking a soda or having a candy bar. I always thought a sandwich on whole wheat bread was a healthy lunch, and I avoided sodas and candy bars. Had I been misled all these years? To make matters worse, I learned that we all fall subject to hidden wheat that's often added to processed foods, chewing gum, prescription drugs, certain cosmetics, toothpaste, and hand cream, to name a few. While Dr. Davis doesn't blame modern wheat as the initial cause of chronic conditions, he presents interesting evidence and reasons to avoid wheat in your diet and products. So, I began using gluten-free makeup. I wasn't going to let the morphine-addictive qualities of wheat worsen my symptoms. I began to understand the once-beloved cookies, cakes, and cereals weren't doing me any favors. However, I still asked the bottom-line question: What is the initial cause of the chronic conditions that we face today?

Jeremiah 33:3 declares, "Call to me, and I will answer you; I will tell to you things great beyond reach of your knowledge." Perhaps, the teacher-recommended chiropractor, Dr. Gram, would have some answers? I drove forty-five minutes to and from the appointments, pleading in prayer for a breakthrough. Dr. Gram was kind, compassionate, and knowledgeable, and he listened. He used blood, urine, and muscle testing to determine problematic areas. His treatment options were plentiful, including chiropractic adjustments, acupuncture, infrared sauna, diet counseling, traction, fascia massage, and supplementation. I saw him a few times a week, for several months, and learned many things: Cellphones take a toll on our immune system; most Americans have a high-fat diet, predisposing us to chronic pain and inflammation; and we are exposed to over eighty thousand man-made chemicals in our water supply. I stopped using our microwave and began using a toaster oven to warm food after his lecture on radiation. One of his clients was a doctor who told him, "I don't know what you are doing, but do your thing!" She sent some of her patients to him.

On the fifth appointment, I struggled to muster up the energy to get dressed and drive to the office. Immediately, he detected that my muscles were off, meaning they weren't giving him any indicators. Teary-eyed, I asked why this kept happening. He responded, "We are generally exposed to a certain level of stress, and if the level is exceeded, then our electrical system shuts down." To perform bodily functions like thinking, moving, and feeling, it's necessary for the nervous system to send signals throughout the body using electrical charges. I felt like my electricity had been shut off from head to toe.

When my hand was hurting the most, a deep, cold, painful numbness and tingling were present. I pictured it as if the cable TV circuits were out, causing black-and-white static on the screen—a block in the electrical signals. The muscle testing part of my appointment resulted in more diet changes: no more grains, rice, buckwheat noodles, chocolate, or coffee. I had to give up my two indulgences: coffee and chocolate. Even though I didn't drink coffee daily, I sure enjoyed the warm, sweet flavor of a decaf cup of java with almond milk. Giving up chocolate for me was like quitting smoking for someone else. I went cold turkey. To compensate for my losses, I bought pecan-flavored coffee beans and put them in a bowl on the kitchen counter, so I could at least smell the aroma until it didn't matter anymore.

At yet another appointment, Dr. Gram revealed the results of my bloodspot fatty acid profile test. One of the numbers was higher than he had ever seen, so he contacted the company to speak with their specialist. It resulted in him announcing, in these words: "You are inflamed!"

No kidding! I thought.

The company had no answers, saying it could've been a false test result. While evidence existed for the bizarre inflammation, there was no solid reason for it. Puzzled by my case, Dr. Gram reached out to a friend in another city, who was also treating a CRPS patient, and who insisted there were emotional components to the disease.

Not this again, I thought.

Alternative and modern medicine are quick to point the "crazy" finger when they don't have answers. There was something else he didn't understand, however. I remembered learning in nursing school that the liver could regenerate itself if needed. I had read that if eighty percent of your liver was removed, it could regenerate itself entirely in three months' time. In addition, due to the liver's unique rejuvenation ability, it is difficult to determine liver damage until it is advanced. In other words, the liver can *conceal* its damage. Erin, the naturopath, once told me that my body wasn't seeing the indicators it needed to see in order to fix itself. *Was my liver involved?*

I also read that castor oil packs, developed by the healer Edgar Cayce, were recommended to clean the liver. These packs are thought to boost the immune system, enhance lymphatic drainage and liver function, remove waste products, stimulate the gallbladder, and increase elimination. I used three of these packs in one month.

To make a pack, I would pour castor oil onto a piece of cotton or wool flannel, fold the flannel into a rectangle, and place it on my right upper abdomen area and around to my back, covering my liver. Then I would lie down for at least thirty minutes (or however long I was able) until I cleaned it off. Afterward, I was wiped out, but I had huge results—military-green poop for forty-five days. No one knew why. All I could think was that the color matched the bile I remembered viewing from our nursing school cadaver. Our livers produce bile to break down the fats we eat. The bile is then stored in the gallbladder. I was eating a high-protein and high-fat diet filled with meats, fish, nuts, and avocados. I must have had a lot of backed-up bile. It seemed my liver was part of my problem.

I shared this piece of the puzzle with a friend. Her acquaintance, who was opening a holistic practice in California, called me to assist with the liver issue. She knew about the castor oil packs but said to be careful, as they penetrate deeply and can release too many toxins, potentially causing the body to feel overwhelmed. She then told me to scream and punch a pillow to get all the anger out of my liver. Really? Where do people come up with this stuff? I wasn't harboring deep-seated anger, except for the anger I felt when people kept telling me my emotions were to blame. My pain and fatigue were more than an outburst of emotional turmoil. Now I understand and have learned that people can harbor anger, given a stagnant liver, yet there was so much more to my story.

I do believe that our emotions play a part in the healing process, yet I had so many physical issues. My hand and leg pain coincided and fluctuated from day to day. My heart palpitations grew more frequent and stronger, lasting for longer time periods, often two hours nightly. In addition, I had hot and cold flashes, low-grade fevers, charley horse cramps in my legs, generalized itching, and dizziness. I tried walking on the treadmill at the gym, but after forty-five minutes, I became extremely dizzy and had to sit down for half an hour before driving home. The day after a junior high fundraiser, I had a "hangover" and pounding headache, not from alcohol but from all the loud music. Chemical fragrances such as perfume, cologne, candles, cleaning supplies, and bath products quickly had me running the other way.

Many days when my symptoms continued and I was tired and frustrated from being isolated and restricted, my children kept me going. In Texas, you can obtain a driver's learning permit at age fifteen, which allows you to drive with a licensed adult. Patrick began driving here and there with me in the car.

On the way back from his orthodontist appointment, I took the liberty to congratulate him. "Last night, you ran an amazing hundred-meter hurdle race. I couldn't believe you broke the freshman high school record. It was easy to spot your long legs out on the track. I'm so proud of you and how hard you practice. It was exciting to watch."

"I couldn't believe it either. It felt great to be in sync with my rhythm. I was determined to improve my time," he said. "But Mom, don't you see how healthy I am? I don't need to change my diet at all," he expressed with youthful invincibility. During the past year, he had probably pushed me the most, demanding answers about the dietary changes I imposed on the family.

"Yes, you are healthy. But I don't want you or your siblings to ever deal with what I've been dealing with. I've reduced wheat and corn products in our home, and friends, coaches, and parents have made comments to me about you guys being faster, more focused, and more energetic. You don't seem to mind the gluten-free pasta and rice. They taste very similar to the regular kind," I pointed out. "I saw your friends making fun of all the organic products in our pantry. I'm sorry about that. They don't understand all the pesticides present in our foods and the harm they do to our bodies," I sympathized.

"Can you just make sure we get to have some of our favorite snacks?" he negotiated.

"Yes, I will. But I'll also have plenty of fruit around too," I voiced. I had to keep seeking answers to educate myself, my family, and others.

"Mom, you should really exercise more often," Patrick announced. "I think it would help you feel better," he continued lecturing. "Coach Nelson says exercise and eating right are the best ways to overcome things," he encouraged. He didn't know that I was doing what my body would allow.

One morning, John woke me up because I had been promising Sarah that I would straighten her hair. After playing hair stylist, I fell back asleep, and John had to drive her to school.

Another morning, in the kitchen Sarah commented, "You are like a different mom."

"How?" I asked, walking over to her and stroking her curly hair.

"You are funny and nice," she delightfully exclaimed, as she grabbed a strawberry from the colander.

"Maybe I am feeling better. What do you think about that?" I asked her while I stirred soup on the stove.

"I don't know, because I am not you," she answered with her eight-year-old wisdom.

"Let's dance," she persuaded, as she grabbed both of my hands.

My head was dizzy as we shook side to side, hand in hand. I looked into her sparkling, long-lashed eyes and perfectly symmetrical features. I thought to myself how lucky I was to have my children. I told her, "You are so precious, my sweet girl!" I was still trying to heal and holding onto hope.

Another morning, Sarah dreamed a genie appeared and offered her a wish. She first wished my hand would be all better, and then she wished for seventy-seven more wishes. What a smart girl! Then we had alone time in the car, traveling to and from soccer practice. (We still have our best discussions in the car.) Her practice was usually a time for me to sit still, taking in the fresh air. It pained me to miss the end-of-the-season parents versus girls practice session, as I sat on the sidelines as an observer.

John told me that he scoured the internet during his work breaks, searching for more healing information. He said he saw glimpses of the old me shining through for a short time in between the darkness. He said it was like scenes from *The Notebook* by Nicholas Sparks. I didn't know it then, but he wanted to *fix* me. Maybe that's how spouses of the chronically ill feel. But they can't fix what they don't understand. He wanted back the woman whom he married. He wondered if a vacation would perk up my spirits, as though I needed a special prize to replace the chaos.

So, we planned a spring break family vacation to Grand Cayman Island. I wasn't sure how I would fare on this trip, but I figured I could have the same symptoms here or there, and I didn't want to let my family down. We were staying in a hotel, so I emailed the concierge ahead of time a list of foods I could eat and a list of those I needed to avoid. I really didn't know what it would be like to depend on a chef for my meals. The head chef came out to meet me the first night. He was trying to understand medically why I wouldn't eat certain foods. I finally told him I had a condition that modern medicine didn't know the cause or the cure of, and that I was trying to handle it holistically.

The head chef shared that he had a friend who'd been diagnosed with liver cancer, which inspired him and his wife to eat organically and to juice fruits and vegetables. He made my dinner in the hotel's indoor kitchen, while the rest of the family ordered from the outside kitchen. I was anxious about not having food readily available for snack purposes. Being supportive, the chef had some baked chicken and organic strawberries and raspberries sent to our room that fit perfectly in the small refrigerator. I could then have a snack at my leisure.

The next morning's breakfast was my most difficult meal, as I was surrounded by a breakfast buffet complete with biscuits, muffins, pancakes, and waffles that my former self would have dived into headfirst. I was almost in tears, not from resisting temptation, but from both having to explain my circumstances and being in those circumstances. The waiter kept bringing me items that I could not eat, until a bowl of delicious cubed mango landed on the table in front of me. The next morning, I found out that one of the sous chefs had gone to the store and bought organic breakfast sausage just for me. It was pink on the inside, however, and I was fearful it contained red pepper or paprika (both nightshades), so I passed on the sausage. Quickly, I decided that, for future travels, I would need access to a kitchen, transportation, and a grocery store carrying organic products, because my health is *my* responsibility and not the responsibility of a hotel chef or restaurant.

John took our kids on a boat tour to snorkel, fish, and swim with stingrays. They kept asking why I wasn't going on the boat tour. I tried to explain to them how movement on a treadmill made me extremely dizzy, and thus, so would the boat. Once again, I had been separated from my family because of my health. On a positive note, however, I was able to take a long walk on the beautiful white sands and bask in the sunshine. But I was thinking of them on the boat and wishing that I was with them.

When we returned home, my brother and nephew came for a visit as my brother had business nearby. One afternoon, I was supposed to meet them for lunch after setting up a teacher luncheon. I couldn't, unfortunately, because I was too exhausted, so I returned home to my bed. Since I was out of capacity, John brought dinner home from a seafood restaurant. I ordered my usual: plain steamed green beans and plain steamed fish. During the night, my pain suddenly escalated beyond measure. The following morning, I was inspired to call the restaurant to ask how the meal was prepared. Usually, this meal did not affect me, but the green beans had been sautéed instead of steamed. The manager then said that the green beans were marinated and cooked in chicken stock, onions, tomatoes, and peppers. I figured this was another nightshade episode. I had been avoiding nightshades since the last time they'd induced an awful migraine. It took two long weeks for the pain to lessen after this episode. I had grown weary of worrying about everything I put in my mouth and worrying about food hurting me. My body was rejecting so many foods, and it was becoming impossible to eat out or trust a restaurant. It felt insane to be living in fear of food. My life was going down the drain, and I needed to find the drain stopper *fast*. I decided it was the final straw—I knew I needed more help.

Every time I returned home from Dr. Gram's office, John would ask, "You bought *more* supplements?" There were changes every week to supplements I should take, how many to take, and how often to take them. It was all very inconsistent, and I found that some supplements made me feel worse. The kind and humble Dr. Gram believed in the "full reveal" labeled supplements that he sold; however, there was no improvement. He taught me that all supplements weren't created equally, and some supplements don't list added ingredients and fillers on their labels. However, he said that the supplements he suggested were clean, used manufacturing quality controls, and met certain regulations. According to an article by Stephanie Watson found on WebMD, supplements are not regulated by the FDA for safety and efficacy before they hit the market. The article suggests choosing supplement brands that are labeled with a third-party quality controls seal from organizations such as NSF International, U.S. Pharmacopeia, Underwriters Laboratory, or Consumer Lab. Even though I was taking many of these clean supplements, my symptoms persisted without an end in sight.

Dr. Gram followed and respected lectures and newsletters by Dr. Levi Mabrey, who was considered a specialist in the field of chiropractic medicine. Dr. Mabrey taught other natural healthcare practitioners the techniques he developed using muscle testing. Dr. Gram knew I was familiar with Dr. Mabrey's nightshade toxicity proficiency, and that I had once tried to make an appointment with him without luck. He told me that "sometimes different docs see different things," and maybe I should contact Mabrey again for an appointment.

So, I decided Dr. Levi Mabrey was the next person I'd seek out for help. At my last appointment with Dr. Gram, his mom and part-time receptionist gave me a gift. She knew I was fearful of my circumstances as she had watched me struggle week to week. She gifted me a devotional book titled *Jesus Calling* by Sarah Young. In the book, there was a devotion for each day of the year. The message on that day stated that we as humans are called "to live by faith, not by sight."

CHAPTER 5

Lyme Disease

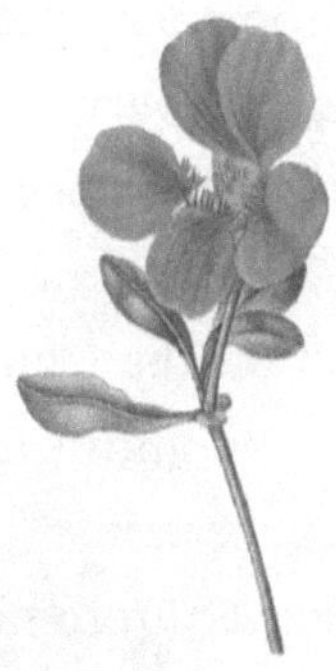

"I'm making an appointment with Dr. Mabrey," I told John one Saturday morning as we sat in our formal living room in our pajamas, catching up on the week.

"What? Don't you think you are jumping the gun? I don't know if I can take off work right now, and what about the kids?" he questioned, thinking I was being erratic.

I stood up to look out the front window into our cul-de-sac. "All I know is what I've been doing with Dr. Gram isn't working. I need to try something else. I know it's another expense, but I don't know what else to do. I'm going with or without you," I proclaimed, before there was any more resistance from him.

A few days later, John woke me up from a nap in our bedroom before taking Evan to basketball practice.

"Amber has dinner ready for y'all," I offered.

"Okay, I'll eat when I get back. I checked my schedule, and I can go with you mid-April to see Dr. Mabrey. My parents said they would stay with the kids while we were gone. My mom told me I couldn't let you go across the country alone," he admitted.

I was terribly nervous to make the call, but I did it anyway. Dr. Mabrey, the chiropractic specialist and nightshade-knowledgeable practitioner, was very serious and short-winded. He made no promises to be able to help me, yet he had agreed to see me *if* I followed his directions. I told him that I was the most compliant patient on the planet and was only eating around twenty things. An appointment was scheduled for ten days later. John was still uncertain of these plans, but I was grateful that he came with me. From his years of traveling for work, he had more experience maneuvering airports, rental cars, hotels, and new cities.

The night before we flew several states away, we had Patrick's end-of-season basketball banquet. I brought my dinner in a little ice chest while everyone else ate the catered food. A friend at the banquet suggested restaurants to us in the area near Dr. Mabrey's office. I knew, however, that their kind suggestions didn't pertain to me. We arranged a rental car and a few nights' stay at a Residence Inn, which came equipped with a full kitchen and plenty of grocery stores nearby.

After the banquet, it was time to snuggle Sarah into bed. She brushed her teeth, then got under her covers. "Dad and I will be gone for a few days. Frannie and Big John will be here with you guys. All your soccer uniforms and clothes are clean." I told her, trying to comfort Sarah with logistics while my thoughts were in disbelief of my predicament. We were only an hour from the well-respected Houston Medical Center, but we were having to take a three-hour flight to seek care. This doctor had been an extra card that I was holding in my hand. In fact, he was my *last* card. *Would he have insight, or would I have CRPS for the rest of my life?*

"I hope the doctor answers all of your prayers," Sarah expressed in her young, innocent way. I hugged her as tight as I could and kissed her all over her beautiful face. My strong, handsome teen boys also told me they hoped the doctor visit went well. Their uniforms and clothes were clean too, even though they were usually responsible for their own laundry. They all deserved their mom back.

As our plane raced down the runway, so did the tears down my cheeks. There was nothing but emptiness inside my soul. I was beyond nervous the following morning for my appointment. A fresh white blanket of snow calmed my nerves, as if a clean slate would define the day. I opted to brush my fears aside and put on the full armor of the Lord's strength as we walked into the doctor's office.

Using muscle testing, Dr. Mabrey said I tested positive for *Borrelia*, the bacteria thought to be transmitted by infected ticks as the cause of Lyme disease. He said I also tested positive for *Bartonella* and *Babesia*, two co-infections commonly found with Lyme disease. He explained that the three pathogens cause different symptoms, and the use of antibiotics had not been one hundred percent successful in Lyme patients because the current antibiotics were unable to kill all three pathogens. He added that some patients have relapses when using the antibiotics, leaving them without curative results and with liver toxicity.

He told us that he worked with the top Lyme doctors in the country, developing new treatment protocols. He sounded knowledgeable and seemed to possess cutting-edge ideas to beat this disease. Dr. Mabrey's passion for detecting and treating Lyme disease was personal, as he was also experiencing Lyme symptoms.

My Lyme disease diagnosis was overwhelming. I didn't know anyone with Lyme disease, and I didn't know anything about it. When we googled how to treat it, every site reported that a few weeks of antibiotics would cure all the symptoms. *Could it be that easy?* Initially, John and I, along with our families, were ecstatic, imagining our lives would be back to normal after just a few weeks, according to the internet. But the internet's information wasn't in sync with Dr. Mabrey's afternoon lecture against the use of antibiotics for Lyme disease. Had we found the needle in the haystack? Had we found answers and a complete cure? Dr. Mabrey verified that I had solanine toxicity syndrome (STS) but offered it may become a permanent problem if one of *his* supplements couldn't get it excreted out of my body. He had discovered my Lyme disease, but how were CRPS, STS, and Lyme disease all related?

Dr. Mabrey, like Dr. Gram, sold high-quality supplements, but Dr. Mabrey went a step further. He worked with a company to create new, clean products he felt surpassed the best testing methods. Since these supplements were safer and cleaner than others, without unnecessary added ingredients, I assumed these supplements could be a good choice to hopefully wash away the pain and fatigue of Lyme disease. Dr. Mabrey handed me some supplements to take that evening before another appointment the next day. That night, I hardly slept, with my body painfully tingling from head to toe, my heart palpitations racing, and my mind wildly circulating with questions. Prior to my second appointment, John and I went to church to pray, as this new process and information were foreign to us. By that point, I could hardly move.

"How are you feeling?" asked the thin, bushy-bearded chiropractor.

"My body is tingling all over, my head is spinning, and I can hardly keep my eyes open. I just want to go back to sleep. It feels like my body went to war," I expressed.

"Well, I overloaded you on pathogen-killing supplements overnight to be able to assess the effects and be sure of the Lyme disease," he explained. In his practice, clinical diagnosis was often necessary because traditional blood tests for Lyme disease were highly inaccurate.

"I wish you lived nearby, but since you don't, I'm going to teach John how to muscle-test you," he remarked.

It was difficult to concentrate, yet we were quickly dependent on this man for instructions. First, he had me lie down on the examination table. Then he proceeded to move my arms in various movements. He showed John that by placing some supplements near my body and pressing on my arm while I resisted, my arm would either weaken or strengthen. If I couldn't hold my arm up when Dr. Mabrey tried to push it down, the supplement was considered to be weakening my arm, and therefore, I shouldn't take it for that round. But if I could hold my arm up when Dr. Mabrey tried to push it down, the supplement was considered to be strengthening my arm, and therefore, I should take it for that round. Per Dr. Mabrey's instructions, John was to muscle-test me three times a day, and we were to keep a log of which supplements I needed and took each time. He told us to look for a pattern, as the key to healing Lyme disease was a rhythm of using supplements to kill the pathogens and supplements to detox them. He estimated I should have a full recovery in six to eighteen months. We had a plan, we had answers, we had an understanding (somewhat), and we had work to do. We needed to return home to regroup and decide on our best course of action.

Family members didn't comprehend going against modern medicine and the internet. One family member yelled at me, insisting I go see a cardiologist, take control of my health before I died, and get some antibiotics ASAP. I had already seen a cardiologist and had disclosed all my heart palpitations. The cardiologist had declared the palpitations I experienced could just be my perception, that they could simply stem from the position of my heart, or that my heart's electrical impulses were taking place at a slightly different angle than normal. My electroencephalogram (EEG) and echocardiogram (EKG) were both normal. He did no further testing and couldn't truly explain the heart palpitations. It felt as if I'd just run in a race, and my heart was pumping quicker and quicker, yet I was sitting or lying still. I knew it was more than my perception. But what I didn't know was if I was going to have permanent heart damage.

Another family member didn't understand why I didn't drop everything and travel to Florida, where a doctor online was claiming to completely heal all of his Lyme disease patients. But there were days when I couldn't make it to the grocery store or even get out of bed. We heard about a friend of a friend who went to see the doctor in Florida. In time, the man returned home in even worse shape and had been depleted of his personal finances.

A third family member insisted that all the answers could be found within me. I dug deep, wondering if I had experienced some trauma or abuse that was holding me back or if some wisdom was residing on my mind's outskirts. Yet, nothing surfaced. Still another well-meaning family member must've thought I was off my rocker and told John I needed an intervention. I was at another crossroads and extremely protective of my worn-down body. I needed more information, and once again, anger fueled my research.

When deciding on the best course of action, I ran into three main problems. The first conflict revolved around treatment. Should I try to find a doctor to prescribe antibiotics to treat Lyme disease, or heed the warning from Dr. Mabrey to bypass the antibiotics and focus on taking his suggested herbal supplements? I chose to start with my local primary doctor. I asked him to order a Lyme disease test, but he was reluctant. He said he'd only seen one Lyme patient with the telltale early sign indicator of a rash on the calf. It is an expanding rash that develops a red ring around an insect bite, giving the appearance of a bull's-eye on a dartboard. Ticks are the insects blamed for Lyme disease. This bull's-eye rash was the second problem existing in the Lyme twilight zone.

Some Lyme disease patients have this rash, while others don't. Doctors insisted that patients with Lyme disease symptoms and/or a positive test without the bull's-eye rash in plain sight must have the bull's-eye rash on their heads where it couldn't be seen. I didn't have the rash in plain sight or on my head, and my primary doc insisted that Lyme was difficult to diagnose. I explained to him it had taken a year of enduring multiple symptoms before I received this diagnosis from someone states away who worked with the top Lyme doctors in the United States. My doctor finally agreed to appease me by giving me a Lyme blood test. It was negative. Such tests, however, were also widely known to produce false positives and false negatives. The Centers for Disease Control and Prevention (CDC) recommends a two-tiered blood test for Lyme disease, known as the Enzyme-Linked Immunosorbent Assay (ELISA) and Western Blot. Yet neither can detect the bacteria thought to cause Lyme disease; they only detect if a patient's body has produced antibodies for it. Those faulty tests were my third problem with the Lyme disease conundrum.

In an effort for more information, I searched my computer for local help. The Texas Lyme Disease Association (TXLDA) popped up on screen. When I clicked on the link in 2013, I was spooked. There was no website, just absolutely *nothing* on the black screen but the words: "Fill in the information and someone will be in touch with you." It was bizarre, yet after I filled in my information, I actually received a phone call from one of the TXLDA vice presidents. She proceeded to tell me her son's

Lyme story. If I remember correctly, her son was bitten by a tick on a Boy Scout trip. He had been on antibiotics for years, and she fed him organically with low carbs and plenty of fruits and vegetables. I don't remember any mention of an actual cure. She rattled off a few Lyme-literate doctors between Texas and Louisiana, but they all seemed to treat the disease with antibiotics, weren't seeing patients anymore, or were hours away.

Even amid the Lyme doctors, there were two different camps: Infectious Diseases Society of America (IDSA) and International Lyme and Associated Diseases Society (ILADS). In short, the IDSA camp stood their ground, stating a short course of antibiotics would heal Lyme patients. The ILADS camp recognized the patients were suffering and fought for the use of long-term antibiotics to help them. I wasn't finding easy answers, but I was finding inconsistencies as we heard more personal stories.

Once my Lyme disease diagnosis was revealed to friends and family, we were informed about numerous different Lyme situations. John spoke with a guy from work whose wife had suffered from Lyme disease twice and found relief with antibiotics. A friend of a friend and her daughter both had Lyme disease symptoms. She didn't have the telltale bull's-eye rash, but her daughter did. She visited Harvard Medical School and had every test possible, all with no results. She took oral antibiotics for a year, but her symptoms persisted. Then she went to a Lyme disease specialist in California who sent her blood samples to the IGeneX lab, however her results were inconclusive. Located in California, the IGeneX lab is a lab specializing in detecting tick-borne illnesses. They use the IGeneX Immunoblot test for Lyme disease, claiming to test for antibodies to more strains of *Borrelia* than the Western Blot test. Her parents were physicians and ordered intravenous (IV) antibiotics for her and her daughter. Eight years later, she noticed she had a bull's-eye rash following an outdoor hike and returned to California for more IV antibiotics. Both she and her daughter continue to have lingering symptoms.

I called a wellness clinic an hour away from my home, seeking treatment and answers. The clinic did not accept my private insurance and treated their patients with supplements. The clinic was run by a married doctor and nurse couple. The nurse divulged she had battled Lyme disease but was cured, although she was dependent on her infrared sauna daily. They had also used the IgeneX lab in California to diagnose Lyme disease, all for a fee of $1,500, not including supplements. I choose not to pursue an appointment. Being dependent on a sauna didn't sound like a cure to me, and I already had supplements to try.

One of Sarah's fourth-grade teachers thought about me over the summer. She was visiting her mom in Vermont and got bitten by a tick on her head while gardening. When she returned to Texas, her primary doctor prescribed her ten days' worth of the antibiotic doxycycline. He explained that, while in New York, he had consulted with a physician who treated patients with Lyme disease under the radar. He told her that most Texas doctors don't treat it, and that it wasn't worth testing because the current tests were inconclusive. At the time, the CDC was adamant about Lyme disease not existing in Texas, although I was receiving the Texas Lyme Disease newsletter.

Sarah's soccer coach and his beautiful wife brought me a rosary from the Vatican. The rosary beads were made from crushed roses, and it smelled wonderful. Their precious gift inspired me to start praying the Rosary several times a week. I usually prayed it in the sauna or during the night when I was awake for hours with pain and heart palpitations. This newly-wed couple was extremely compassionate. One day after Sarah's soccer practice, he told me his brother in Connecticut had Lyme disease and had been treated with intramuscular injections for about six months with good results. His brother had presented with the bull's-eye rash and was aware that he'd been bitten by a tick. His story seemed to be a typical acute case of Lyme. My case, however, was chronic. When a Lyme disease diagnosis is delayed, the illness can progress to late-stage Lyme disease, presenting with ongoing and widespread multi-systemic symptoms. I was in late-stage Lyme disease, making it more difficult to treat, and antibiotics usually did not help.

Regular physicians in Texas weren't familiar with diagnosing or treating Lyme disease, so I was instructed to seek out a Lyme-literate medical doctor (LLMD). LLMDs have kept a low profile because their licenses were being pulled for prescribing long-term antibiotic therapy. It's no secret that antibiotics pose risks like liver toxicity, immune suppression, and antibiotic resistance to further infections. But people have suffered greatly with Lyme symptoms, and these physicians have put their careers on the line to help them.

People were getting sick, and real answers and real cures weren't available, unless one had an acute case with minor symptoms and/or a bull's-eye rash. This disease is riddled with contradictions. I knew that I had to keep searching, so once again I began reading for a better life. I read several books about Lyme disease. *Cure Unknown* by Pamela Weintraub was by far the most in-depth literary work on the topic. It was evident that she was on the frontlines of the disease both personally and professionally. As a science journalist, Weintraub never imagined her entire family would be struck by the mystery illness of controversial Lyme disease when they moved to fresh-aired and wooded Chappaqua, New York.

If you really want to understand how the evolution of Lyme disease was scientifically investigated, *Cure Unknown* is the book for you! I truly don't know how Weintraub wrote it while battling her own brain fog and fighting for the health of herself, her two sons, and her husband. Her book gave me an honest, grave view of the disease, as the word "relapse" was repeatedly mentioned. On the last page of her book, she wrote, "I waited years for a better ending, but it never came. Year after year more Lyme patients were misdiagnosed, mistreated, then meanly hung out to dry." This disease keeps people running on an imaginary hamster wheel as they try out assorted ways to heal. Currently, the CDC still only recommends ten to fourteen days of antibiotics, leaving those with long-term symptoms without care and leaving primary doctors without options to help their patients.

Learning the disease's origins is important when choosing a treatment plan. In 1975, a concerned mother named Polly Murray recognized an alarming number of juvenile rheumatoid arthritis cases that had cropped up in her hometown of Lyme, Connecticut. Numerous kids were walking with the assistance of crutches, along with her own children. Murray contacted the Connecticut Department of Public Health but was told there was nothing they could do. In a neighboring town, another concerned woman, Judith Mensch, called the Department of Public Health as well as the CDC. She learned about a CDC program for young doctors to learn epidemiological training, studying locations and incidence of disease.

Dr. Allen Steere, a rheumatologist at Yale University, worked in the CDC program. He had begun seeing many patients in the area but *did not find bacteria* in joint fluids, so he thought the disease might be *caused by a virus*. Known as the pioneer in Lyme disease, Steere deemed this new disease "Lyme arthritis." It wasn't until 1982, when Dr. Burgdorfer, an entomologist, discovered a spirochete bacterium in the gut of ticks. Since then, the cause of Lyme disease has been blamed on the bacteria named *Borrelia burgdorferi*.

In my research, I discovered how those who were supposed to be protecting us—who were supposed to be holding our medical welfare in their best interest—had been working merely for themselves. In the book *Beating Lyme* by Constance A. Bean and Lesley Ann Fein, the charades surrounding a Lyme vaccine called Lymerix were exposed. Weintraub, along with Bean and Fein, explained in detail the failure of Lymerix, which was pulled off the market due to a lawsuit, after harming vaccinees. In the first year after the vaccine was on the market, there were 298 adverse reactions to the vaccine, and ten percent of those injected reported chronic arthritis. Other complaints included flu-like symptoms, aches and pains all over their bodies, auto-immune diseases that were suddenly triggered, a pounding heart, depression, chronic fatigue, balance problems, brain fog, dizziness, sensitivity to light and sound, and more.

In my Lyme education, I became woke and frustrated, as I learned about the collaborations between the pharmaceutical companies, government agencies, universities, and the private sector that each profited from all things Lyme-related. Weintraub, Bean, and Fein said the problem began with the passing of the Bayh-Dole Act in 1980, which gave permission for universities, their faculty members, and individuals to patent discoveries made with federally funded research grants. Bean and Fein specified there were at least three drug companies, one university, health departments, scientists, and physicians who had shares in the Lymerix vaccine. Also, Weintraub explained the CDC, National Institutes of Health (NIH), and the Department of Defense (DoD) owned partial rights to revenue from more than a third of the fifty-six U.S. patents specifically important for Lyme disease vaccines and tests. My father-in-law has always said, "Where there is confusion, there is profit." I realized that money landed in some pockets, while people continued to be sick. I still wondered, however, was the cure still unknown?

With the problems, conflicts, and agendas surrounding Lyme disease in the medical field, I felt even more confident that I should be on an alternative Lyme protocol. I felt I wouldn't be hurting myself with loads of antibiotics. Maybe Dr. Mabrey's advice was just what I needed to overcome the struggle. My bedside table was covered in Dr. Mabrey's supplements. John thoughtfully made me a spreadsheet to keep track of which supplements I took each day and periodically emailed it to Dr. Mabrey since he lived out of state. Dr. Mabrey suggested I visit a new chiropractor located a half-hour drive from home. My first appointment with the new doctor was disappointing because he found new issues and recommended that I take much higher doses of some of my current supplements in addition to new ones.

"*More* supplements?" chimed John, right on cue.

I had hoped there would've been more progress. The new chiropractor explained that treating Lyme disease takes time. Hypothetically, he said, if you set aside six minutes to clean six items in the kitchen each night, but one night you have a party with eighty-four people in attendance, you would never catch up on all those dirty dishes. Meaning that the immune system can only fight off so much in one day. When overloaded, it takes a long time and the right tools for it to get the job done. *Did I have the right tools? What's overloading my immune system?*

Those higher doses took a toll after a week. I had planned to take Sarah shopping that Saturday. She had outgrown her clothes, and all her pants were high-waters. But I had no energy and had been tingling from head to toe, in addition to experiencing persistent heart palpitations and dizziness. That same day, a friend texted an invite for Sarah and me to join her and her daughter on a bike ride to enjoy the cooler September temps. I didn't even step outside, taking a three-hour nap instead. John tried to wake me for Saturday evening church, but I couldn't get out of bed. The next day, I tossed the higher doses aside and returned to my original plan. All I knew was that my family needed whatever I could give them, and the extra doses certainly weren't helping.

Some days, I stayed in bed and only got up to go to the bath-room or to the kitchen for meals. I went to the ER to rule out blood clots because the pain in my calves was outlandish. An ultrasound of my legs revealed no blood clots, and the doctor asked if I wanted pain medicine. Why were doctors so willing to prescribe pain meds? Those narcotic pain meds didn't help with this kind of pain anyway. An ER nurse encouraged me to let my primary care physician know about my ER visit. I told her it wasn't necessary to inform them because they didn't understand chronic persistent Lyme disease, nor did they know how to treat it.

I guess education on the truth about Lyme disease is a dream of mine, I wrote in my journal. *I wish there were better testing methods for Lyme.* Having Lyme was like being in a house that looks perfectly normal, even warm and inviting. However, when the beautifully painted walls are demolished, you see the structural damage, faulty wiring, and corrosive leaks creating an unsafe environment. With Lyme, you must look beyond the surface to find the truth—the toxins creating chronic illness.

I couldn't comfort John's frustrations with my taking more supplements. I had to deal with my own frustrations and perse-vere. Trial and error was the only way, as I kept being reminded to trust this alien path. I was under spiritual training to build a grateful mindset and a firm foundation, where life's storms could not cause disruption despite circumstances. My friend Susan, who was battling diabetes in addition to Lyme, once told me, "Physical impairments are spiritual journeys." I had never thought of it that way.

CHAPTER 6

Big, Bright, Beautiful Flowers

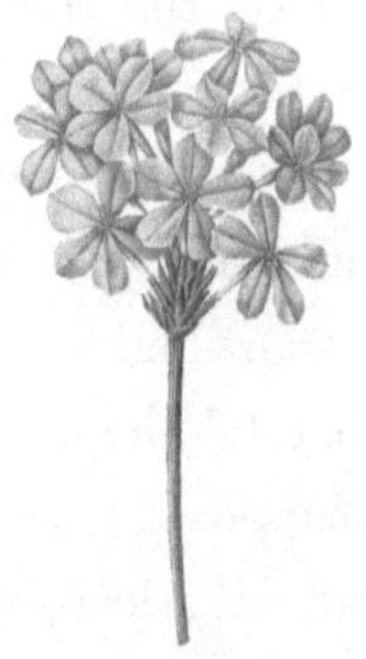

WHEN I WAS YOUNG, I collected quotes that inspired me. I journaled them in a little red book. Of course, this was before the internet, so we couldn't retrieve the written word 24/7. I wrote these quotes down because they carried power, and I wanted the words and their power close to me. This one comes to mind now:

> "Your task is to build a better world," God said.
>
> I answered, "How? This world is such a large place, so complicated now, and I am so small and useless, there's nothing I can do."
>
> But God in all His wisdom said, "Just build a better you."
>
> —UNKNOWN

I suffered from several controversial and misunderstood issues: Lyme disease, solanine toxicity syndrome, and CRPS. How was I going to turn this around? How was I going to get my life back with no traditional medical assistance? When John was in a bind, he would say, "You've got to *reverse* that!" How was I going to reverse all of this? I realized I had to build a better me—it's what I had to do!

One morning, as I sat on the couch in the living room, Sarah rushed downstairs in her pink nightgown to tell me about her dream. As she fiddled with another loose tooth, she said, "I put my tooth under my pillow, but the Tooth Fairy didn't come. I went downstairs and found a huge pile of money with a note saying, 'For Sarah.' Then, under the pile, I found a magic potion, which was supposed to cure Lyme disease. Mom, then you drank the potion, fell asleep, and woke up completely cured!!"

"Well, I can't wait to meet this Tooth Fairy!" I responded. Analyzing her dream, I remembered we had forgotten about the mystical duties. I was thankful Sarah's imagination was still thriving as I hugged her "good morning." Every bit of encouragement was appreciated because the supplements I took seemed to increase my symptoms. I endured the pain because I was taught when the pathogens were killed, neurotoxins were released, causing pain and discomfort—a Jarisch-Herxheimer reaction. It was a one step forward, two steps back protocol.

Days and nights were still unpredictable. I was thrilled to make it to our friend's summer soiree, but I stayed up later than usual. That night, I was riddled with ongoing symptoms, so the following day, I had no energy to leave the house. On the bright side, I watched the Wimbledon men's quarter-final matches from bed. Then the next day I felt better, and I went to use the infrared sauna, to the store, and to a game for one of the kids. Once I had three full night's sleep in a row, so I'd think to myself, *I'm getting better*, until the following night, when I was awake for hours with ongoing heart palpitations. They were so intense that I thought my heart was going to pop right out of my chest and walk away as if it had a life of its own.

Another time, there were four days in a row where I managed mild symptoms and was able to walk Fluffy farther on the path past the lake near our home. *Am I rising from the torment? Am I coming out of the darkness?* I'd dare to ponder. On the fourth after-noon, I had a haircut. My hairdresser already knew not to use her hairspray on my head, but once she used hair gel and you guessed it—a horrible migraine, another step backward.

After going to the grocery store in preparation for celebrat-ing Frannie's birthday and watching the LSU football game, I rushed home for John to muscle-test me. I was about to fall asleep on my bed but knew I needed to take my supplements. As I got a glass of water in the kitchen to take them, I felt lightheaded. I darted for the couch before fainting. Brain fog washed over me, along with the chills and sweats. Three days later, I could barely get out of bed to tell my kids goodbye as they left for school. Thoughtfully, Evan found me back in bed to tell me goodbye. My head was so heavy and dizzy. The next day, I was gladly able to take Fluffy for a walk. It had been weeks since our last walk. *Was I rising from the ashes?* At the sound of the word "walk," her ears perked, tail wagged, and her tongue popped out. She barked and jumped from couch, to chair, to ottoman. She could not contain herself! We walked about a mile, then she headed for her bowl of water as I went to take a shower. As I was getting dressed, I nearly fainted on my closet floor. I finally made it to bed, where I had to rest for an hour before carrying on with my day.

I had vertigo, nausea, constipation, muscle spasms, low-grade temperatures, headaches, neck stiffness, swollen lymph nodes, shortness of breath, and so on. My ears hurt when I slept on them, and my right hand hurt the most out of all my limbs, which were possessed with peripheral neuropathy. Often, my legs hurt too much to walk upstairs to tell the kids goodnight. Sometimes, I did anyway. Other times, I couldn't take another step. Ordinarily, I was functioning at fifty percent or less. I took naps in between driving the kids around and going to the grocery store. With the onslaught of all those symptoms, I dreamed of being a "real girl" as Pinocchio dreamed of being a real boy someday. When I had a few good days in a row, I became cautiously optimistic that the darkness was lifting, and then the bad days would trickle in and wash away my hope. I thought maybe I had turned the corner, but I hadn't . . . over and over and over again.

John was doing double duty at home and at work, during the weekdays and the weekends. Early to work, he made sure Patrick was awake to catch the bus or drive to school. Being the breadwinner, John came home one day and announced our health insurance cost had dropped twenty percent. The year before, we'd noted CRPS as a preexisting condition, and they inflated our rates by twenty percent to cover the cost usually spent by CRPS patients. Unfortunately, after doing the math, I realized that we had spent over $10,000 out-of-pocket. I hoped this high price tag would someday help me and all sufferers with chronic symptoms. We were grateful to receive the insurance payment cut because the supplements were an ongoing out-of-pocket expense.

John must have been feeling the pressure to meet all the demands of his new company. On top of his responsibilities, he was adjusting conference calls and meeting times to muscle-test me midday. I'd coordinate with him via text: "What time will you be home to test me?"

He'd answer with: "I'll be there at 12:30," "I can't make it today," or "I'll come after my 10:00 A.M. meeting." He knew I began feeling poorly as it got closer to testing time, and that often I felt better after taking the supplements. He made an effort day after day. It was his part in this process.

Sometimes, I traveled with him to the boys' basketball tournaments. We were tethered by our constant battle with chronic Lyme disease. When it was time to return home from one of Patrick's tournaments in Dallas, I woke up with head pain that I had never known. It was in truth so bad that I thought I might have to be life-flighted home. After more supplements and more sleep, I finally was able to tolerate the four-hour ride. For one of Evan's tournaments in Austin, we stayed in a different hotel than the team since we needed a kitchen. He didn't say anything, but I knew that Evan would've preferred to stay with the team. It would've been more fun, I'm sure! I was grateful for my earplugs, as the tournament's noise of the balls bouncing, hands clapping, spectators shouting, whistles blowing, and buzzers ringing out was simply too much for me.

It was fun to watch my boys play basketball, though. Their development mentally, socially, and physically was on display on the courts. They were smart players and very passionate. Watching them play was an insight into their world, and I didn't want to miss any more buzzer-beater wins if I could help it. I was particularly glad that I attended this tourney because Evan took a spill on the court, and I heard it from the stands. I saw his reaction and knew it was the end of his season. We bought crutches and supplies at the local drug store. We went with the team to Barton Springs, a popular swimming site in Austin, Texas. An underground spring fills the local reservoir with very cool water, which was good for Evan's ankle. I sat there over-stimulated and worried about Evan, so I prayed silently as the splashing around us continued. Evan then found a shiny penny right by my foot. All would be alright, eventually. He had the first of two ankle surgeries soon thereafter.

The boys still didn't realize how fragile my body was. They teased me about not exercising or cooking. They didn't know that I was using the sauna while they were at school. They didn't know that I had tried exercising but could only tolerate walking. I wasn't going to the gym or eating out, either. Occasionally, a friend would stop by, but mostly people wanted to meet for lunch or go to dinner. I/We usually declined, so the invites declined as well. I was alone a lot—alone with my thoughts and alone with God. I had plenty of thoughts about how and why I was supposed to write this book. I also had plenty of thoughts about me being a drain on my family, in addition to thoughts of needing to leave this Earth when the pain came in electrifying waves, time and time again.

Lyme disease was too confusing and debilitating to even find a support group because everyone had varying symptoms and protocols. There were (and still are) several Facebook groups with people seeking out doctors, desperate to heal themselves or their children. When I became impatient or just needed to talk, I journaled. My journal always listened.

Every day I turned to my brown-covered *Jesus Calling* devotional book for inspiration. My faith was blossoming to a new level as I felt more and more dependent on God's unconditional love. Some days, I had positive energy and breathed in the goodness around me from people and from nature. I became better able to handle the bad days when I was called to surrender to a stay-at-home or bedridden day. Often, my legs felt like I had just finished running a marathon, but I hadn't run in well over a year. When my dishwasher broke, I stood at the sink for hours, washing dishes until my legs were pounding. Those were the days that I lay down, with the TV remote, my cellphone, my iPad, and research books scattered about on the bed. Fluffy was always by my side as well, happy to have someone to sleep next to. I counted on *Today with Kathie Lee and Hoda* to take me out of my bedroom into whatever positive news they shared to brighten my day and make me laugh. I listened to the song "Help Me Find It" by Sidewalk Prophets, which helped me find peace when I needed to be still.

I constantly refilled my hope basket with instructions like these from *Jesus Calling*:

> When things seem to be going all wrong, stop and affirm your trust in Me. Calmly bring these matters to Me, and leave them

in My capable hands. Then, simply do the next thing. Stay in touch with Me through thankful, trusting prayers, resting in My sovereign control.

For me, this particular quote summarized the four overall messages of the book: trust, putting things in God's hands, praying prayers of thanksgiving, and resting in His control. It was my hot air balloon ride to a better day.

Continually finding the pennies reminded me to trust. I mentally and figuratively placed myself in His hands during my pain episodes. I created a meditation prayer, envisioning Mother Mary enfolding me in a blanket and rocking me in a quiet house. Another meditation centered on Jesus carrying me up a stairway to heaven and placing me in God's right hand, where I absorbed holy comfort and strength. In the same fashion, I placed anything that was a burden in His hands. Sometimes, I needed to be extra close to God's divinity, so I'd picture myself next to His heart, in His shirt pocket, as if He wore a shirt.

Jesus Calling taught me gratitude was the best way to reach God's heart. Even on my worst days, there was always something to be grateful for, such as my comfortable bed or the bright, warming sunshine. I was digesting the book's lessons, but I hadn't *fully* rested in His control. I realized that I had consistently set myself up for failure as timelines came and went without progress, dumping doom and gloom into my lap. *Jesus Calling* invited me to partake in timelessness alongside the divine realm. I had to release the demands of time and focus on His presence, where peace was initiated.

I thought about my aunt, who had lost her home in Louisiana and her condo in Mississippi during Hurricane Katrina. "What are you going to do now?" I asked her.

She replied, "I don't make plans anymore, I leave it up to God!" Her faith was something I wanted to mimic. She wasn't concerned with where her head would hit the pillow; she just knew it would.

One day after picking up Sarah in her school's car line, she asked, "Mom, are you feeling better today? I found a penny in my backpack!"

"Today is a good day for me, sweetheart, but it will take time for me to heal completely," I reassured her.

"I'm mad at God!" she blurted.

"Why are you mad?" I inquired.

"I'm mad because He isn't answering my prayers! I don't know if He can hear me?"

"I assure you, your prayers are heard, Sarah. God has so many angels in his kingdom, and you even have a guardian angel who is with you always. You are loved beyond measure! We are supposed to keep praying and keep trusting that our prayers will be answered at just the right time," I replied, conscientiously recognizing this teaching moment. I was never mad at God; I *needed* Him. My frustrations lay with our healthcare system, but I was learning to rest in His control.

I wanted to attend Patrick's basketball game an hour away but felt awful, so I went to rest in the sauna and then felt well enough to make the trip. I saw Patrick's new team, met his new coach, then sat with my friend, Hannah. Our sons had become very good friends, and she had always been a faithful inspiration. She kindly asked how I was doing. I was coherent and brave enough to tell her I had been spending three to four days weekly in bed for many months. Usually, I responded with a vague answer, but I began realizing people might understand Lyme disease better if I gave more precise answers. She was shocked by my answer and told me that I wasn't complaining enough. I thought to myself, *I have been extremely too tired to complain.* She intuitively noted that I must be lonely. Yes, I told her I felt like I was on house arrest. She kindly offered to come over and keep me company and then asked how she could help further. I acknowledged she was already helping with the kids' carpool and didn't realize what a huge help it was. What I didn't say, however, was that on bad days, I wasn't good company. When I returned home, I got back in bed for the rest of the day.

A week later, Hannah emailed me a story about surrendering to God's control. There was a pastor who'd become severely ill, which resulted in his absence from his church duties for two years. A woman came to see the pastor and demanded time with him. He sent her a note saying,

> It is by His will I am in this strait place; in that I will rest. He will keep me here in His love and give me the grace in this trial to behave like His child. In His good time, He can bring me out again. How and when, He knows. I am here by God's appointment, In His keeping, Under His training and For His time.

I suppose the woman dropped her demands. This story encouraged me to hang on tight.

I held on to the possibility that I could heal *and* get my

life back. Patrick, who had always had a knack for science, showed me Isaac Newton's third law of motion while doing his homework one night. Newton's third law states that for every action in nature, there is an equal and opposite reaction. I processed that, if I fell and broke my wrist, which caused my body to go haywire, then there would be an equal and opposite reaction—a return to health. I was hoping that following Dr. Mabrey's muscle-testing instructions and taking supplements would be the key. Time would certainly tell. I didn't know if the supplements were working, but somehow, I felt worse when I was off of them.

We saw signs of occasional improvement here and there. Over the summer, we had a wonderful week at the beach—my happy place. We rented a house with a full kitchen, and a grocery store with organic foods was located nearby. I had John there to muscle-test me three times a day and my supplements, scrubbing therapy board, and bed were nearby. Our kids were happy, and John and I were both relaxed. I didn't remember having a meaningful conversation with my children the previous summer, when I was always sleeping and petrified.

I finally felt more engaged with my family. The boys began to divulge more details about their lives. Evan often asked me to bring him to school instead of riding the bus, and I frequently collected Patrick after school or practice. I treasured uninterrupted time alone with my boys in the car because it was rare. It was amazing what I had learned during those few minutes! Patrick and his girlfriend finally made their relationship official, and Evan knew whom he wanted to ask as his date for homecoming—all news to me! One night, after Sarah went to bed, John and I ended up in the kitchen with the boys. I was awake at 9:40 P.M.! John was standing at the sink, cleaning the dinner dishes. Facing John, I was sitting on a barstool and having a late dinner. Patrick and Evan had emerged from their rooms to make their school lunches for the next day.

"Are y'all finished with homework?" I asked.

"Ma, I've probably done enough," Evan casually said.

"What do you mean 'probably'?"

"I don't need to do any more algebra II problems; I got it down, and I already read the CliffsNotes for my English test tomorrow," he explained.

"Dude, how about you read the book?" Patrick spoke, his eyes rolling.

"How about you back off?" Evan joked, as he lunged playfully toward Patrick. Right then, Fluffy propped herself up to attention from a deep sleep. She sensed the thrill and the oncoming chase. Suddenly, the boys were off, running after each other, round and round through the kitchen and the living room in a circle, engaging little Fluffy at warp speed. She barked and barked in an effort to take part in the play, possibly to protect someone or merely be heard. We weren't sure what was happening, but it certainly was a well-known Kelly pastime. Soon, the boys were on top of each other, laughing, as Fluffy howled. This was *normal*—all of it was being a part of our home—part of having physical teenage boys, brothers.

"You were up late tonight and coherent. You weren't like that last year," John remarked after he brushed his teeth. It was a simple yet stellar moment.

Unfortunately, I had found out my ladies' gym was closing its doors, and I would no longer have access to the sauna I'd grown to love. That sauna had given me energy, improved my circulation, and was deeply detoxing as I sweated away heavy metals and other toxins present in my body. It was a must-have for my therapy! So, we bought an infrared dry sauna for our home and kept it in the garage. When it arrived, John took a half day off from work to put it together because he knew it made me feel better and wanted it to be available for me. I had already gone a week without it and was miserable. That's love, people!

The owner of the gym, Shari, was always in a spiritual flow and shared with me how God was working in her life. One morning, she prayed to sell an item, and in thirty minutes it was sold. While that prayer had been answered quickly, everyone knows that other prayers may take time, with God's wisdom championing our own.

I went on one final trip to the gym to use the sauna. After completing my session, Shari asked, "Deborah, would you be open for my daughter, Ashley, and me to pray with you and lay hands on you? Ashley and her husband, Chris, are in town for a wedding and are helping us disband the business. They do missionary work and are gifted with healing prayers."

"Of course!" I answered quickly. I met with the owner and her daughter the very next morning. As I walked into the gym, I saw quite a different atmosphere than I was used to seeing. Boxes were lying about, equipment was missing, and extension cords were haphazardly placed here and there. Shari introduced me to Ashley, then stepped aside as I stood with this peaceful young woman in a corner of the room.

"Hi, I'm Ashley," she began, as she shook my hand. "My husband saw you here yesterday, and he asked me to give you a message. He wants you to know God is *closer* to you than He has ever been. He has been carrying you through the hard times." They knew nothing about me! What an incredible message from a near-stranger!

She continued, "This morning I prayed over the message God intended for me to give you. Then I received a picture of a desert with several big, bright, beautiful flowers *blooming*! I feel it means that in the midst of the suffering and hard times, God has been shifting things around."

"Oh, Ashley, I feel my life has been turned upside down!" I replied.

"He has been pulling things out of your life and replacing those things with what He wants in your life—things that you need in your life. And at just the right time, you will see the blossoms," she rejoiced.

Shari then appeared in a ready position to lay hands on me. Ashley, Shari, and I stood huddled with our heads touching and arms hugging. Ashley began, "Thank you, God, for the struggles You have laid before Deborah. We ask for *complete* healing of her brokenness. We ask You to fill her with strength to use her experience to help others. Also, we ask You to thwart off any resistance that may present itself in the future."

Shari then added, "Thank you, God, for our newfound friendship. As we've been witnessing together each day this week, Your power intervening in the closing of our business. I, too, ask you to heal Deborah's body *completely*, so that she may be renewed with new life."

Holy moly! I had never had someone "lay hands on me." I figured it was just as simple as prayer, yet it was extra powerful. By that point, I was sobbing at the thought of *complete* healing! Complete healing would be a true miracle—a miracle as close to flowers blooming in the dry desert.

It was my turn to speak. I had to say something. "Thank you, God, for the strength to endure these obstacles and learn more and more along the way. Thank you for lighting my path with these deeply compassionate women and other people and prayers needed for each step." Suddenly, from the depth of my inner core, a great sadness erupted, as I relived the years' worth of isolation that I had felt and the brave face I had tried to wear for the sake of my family. It finally spilled entirely out of me. I was completely overwhelmed by the love pouring out of these women on my behalf.

Afterward, I went to the Christian bookstore to get Patrick a token for his car since he was a new driver and it was his sixteenth birthday. While shopping there, something else caught my eye: a devotional book by Sarah Young titled *Jesus Today*, this time with a blue cover. I read the introduction, and much to my surprise, I discovered that the author had Lyme disease and the same two co-infections I also had, and that her book was dedicated to her nephew named Patrick Kelly. *What are the odds?* After reading the introduction, I turned the page and read Isaiah 43:19: "See, I am doing a new thing! Now it springs up; do you not perceive it? I am making a way in the desert and streams in the wasteland."

I thought to myself, *God is near, and I have never heard Him so clearly before.* Then and there, I understood the vision of the desert and the big, bright, beautiful flowers blooming. God has toiled me like a garden. He has removed the weeds, turned my soil, watered me, and fertilized me. He has taken away people, foods, and the independent person I used to be. He has filled me with a complete dependence on Him, as He continues to hold me during the purification process.

HE IS MAKING A WAY!

CHAPTER 7

Do Something

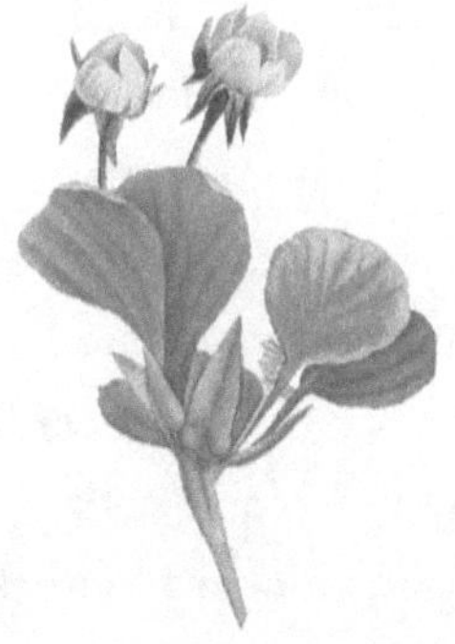

THE WAY TO HEAL was unclear yet. My brain fog was real. During her homework, Sarah asked me how to spell the word *characteristics*. I couldn't help her without using my phone. Then, a previous neighbor walked in the side door of our new home nearby.

She asked, "Deborah, how can I help? What can I do?" She is the kindest, funniest, and most easy-going person to be around. She was someone I felt completely comfortable with. Someone who didn't play games and didn't put on airs. Her curly ash-blonde hair, glasses, and earthy vibe were a welcomed sight. But I just sat there, in a chair, looking out of the window. I heard her words and was happy to see her, but somehow, I couldn't formulate ideas, decisions, or sentences. I couldn't think through creating a to-do list, which was once a favorite addiction. My brain wasn't running on all cylinders. My neighbor paused there, waiting for a response. I remained seated with a blank look on my face, waiting for the words to come to mind, but they didn't. My brain simply wasn't working. She left, and I went to bed. I'd try to reach out to her another time. I knew my health issues were far from normal—far from home.

I continued my doctor-appointment hopping in town, seeking answers to my health. One day, I developed a strange rash on my legs after I was out in the sun. Matching rash images from Google revealed livedo reticularis. In short, it's a dilation of capillary blood vessels and stagnation of blood within the vessels. Another condition associated with the rash is called polycythemia vera (PV), a blood cancer in which the bone marrow makes too many red blood cells, white blood cells, and/or platelets, resulting in thicker blood that can cause clotting, heart attack, stroke, or deep vein thrombosis. *Did I have cancer?* I told my primary care physician about all my symptoms.

"The tingling and numbness in your hands and feet are probably due to stress," he remarked with a straight face, giving me an honest answer as far as he was concerned.

I knew better. My issues were much more complicated. I couldn't help but smile at him and wonder how many times a day he blamed a symptom on stress.

"Let's do some lab work. I may refer you to a neurologist to rule out multiple sclerosis."

Again, my lab results were all within normal limits, and the special blood test used as a diagnostic tool for PV came back negative. I then saw a hematologist for further explanation, but she suggested I take over-the-counter iron supplements. The technician said my blood was so thick that she had difficulty filling the vial. However, the hematologist said my labs looked good, except for my low iron levels, and that I was perfectly fine. *Really?* I took the iron supplements and ate foods high in iron, including meat, yet my iron levels didn't increase. I avoided nuts, oils, and avocados to lower my fat intake. I didn't consider how much fat was in the beef, even in the low-fat beef I'd been consuming in plentiful amounts. Yet, I remained anemic with thick blood.

Per a friend's suggestion, I visited a doctor specializing in chelation therapy to rid the body of heavy metals. I'd read Lyme disease couldn't be cured unless you rid your body of heavy metals. Dr. Mabrey had warned me against traditional chelation techniques because he saw the treatment often resulted in people having irreversible kidney, lung, liver, or heart damage. I wanted a second opinion. However, this new private doctor ignored my chelation request and suggested I take hormones to boost my energy. His treatment was expensive, so I visited my gynecologist, who prescribed the low doses of bioidentical hormones that were much cheaper.

Per another suggestion, I saw a neurologist and thought about requesting an MRI to determine if I had brain lesions like those found in other Lyme and multiple sclerosis (MS) patients. The neurologist, however, wouldn't get near me, staying across the room and insisting she did not (and would not) treat me for Lyme disease. She did order an MRI, but I decided I didn't want to expose myself to the radiation as I was already on treatment. So even if I had the MRI, my treatment wouldn't have changed.

I visited massage therapists, reflexologists, and church healing services, along with numerous other places, searching for healing. I longed to feel well, to eat whatever I wanted, and go wherever I wished. I longed to be set free from my burdens. I had no idea what our out-of-pocket expenses equaled at that point.

Three months passed, six months passed, and finally a year passed without reprieve. John and I flew across the country again for our second meeting with Dr. Mabrey.

"Hi, Dr. Mabrey, how are you?" I asked as we walked into his new office.

"I'm okay these days, better with some symptoms and worse with others," he informed. "Let's have you lie on the table, so we can muscle-test you," he instructed as he jumped into business.

During the testing phase, he asked, "How have you been feeling?"

"A lot like you," I replied. "I have all the same symptoms, but new ones have emerged, and some are getting really bad. My legs are taking the brunt. I've been having charley horses and wobbly legs. Sometimes, it feels like a knife has punctured my calf, or my thighs feel raw and achy as if my muscles were tied in a million knots. My daughter gets frustrated when I keep scratching my legs, but my itching can be intolerable. My heels hurt when I lie in bed, and the burning numbness and tingling in my legs and arms are horrendous. Do you have any of these issues?" I wondered.

"My issues are different," he replied, as he focused on the muscle testing.

"Dr. Mabrey, honestly, sometimes I feel like a dog needing to be put to sleep. Those flares can be so intense, like I would catch on fire easily if someone lit a match nearby. You know, one of my chiropractors had a Lyme patient they treated for five years without resolution, and now she can no longer walk. Am I going to be wheelchair bound? I'm so afraid to lose my legs!"

"How's your balance?" he inquired.

"I keep running into walls, so my balance isn't very good. Every time I empty the dishwasher, I break a glass or a plate. And I keep having fainting spells. My sense of direction has gone amiss. I couldn't find my way to a distant gym for Evan's basketball game or to a neighbor's house ten minutes away to get Sarah from a friend's house. If I drive across a highway overpass, I clinch the steering wheel because I feel like I'm going to fall to the ground. So weird, huh?" I blurted out.

"Any other problems?" he questioned.

"Um, let's see. Yes, I often feel like I still have the flu with achy joints. My night sweats are soaking through two nightgowns a night, but I'm *always* freezing cold, even wearing flannel in the scorching Houston summertime. Are your senses sensitive? I cannot tolerate artificial fragrances, loud noise, or bright lights. I'm always wearing sunglasses, and now I have to wear noise-cancelling headphones to Evan's high school football games," I complained.

"I do have some sensitivities. Do those headphones really cancel the noise?" he asked.

"They really do! Great invention," I advertised. After thirty minutes of moving my arms around, we asked how I was doing, and what he was finding.

He said, "I am disappointed to find so many pathogens. But at the same time, you have potential for more progress." He then added yet a new supplement to my list to take (John was thrilled), found heavy metals in my system and in my makeup, discouraged having root canal removals by a biological dentist as he'd never seen the intervention improve anyone's health, told me to lower the amount of beef and seafood I ingested, and suggested getting a Rife machine.

"What's a Rife machine?" we asked.

"It's a machine that emits electromagnetic frequency waves to delete diseased cells. I've weeded out several Rife machines and suggest one made by a gentleman in New York. He builds them himself and has cured his wife of Lyme."

It sounded promising, so we ordered our own Rife machine, incorporated it into our life, and carried on with all the muscle testing and multiple supplement ingestion. Later, we found out that the man's wife was still dependent on Rife treatments to get through her day.

As time passed, I did overcome some obstacles. I could open a water bottle, I no longer needed my steering wheel knob to help me drive, and I was finished with my scrubbing board therapy after eighteen months. I credited our home infrared sauna and continued doing the hand therapy movements I had learned. I could finally move and use my wrist when the pain was low. However, there were other physical, emotional, and social issues that I had to face.

Overall, I wanted to be understood and heard in the worst way. My parents felt helpless and asked if they could do anything. I told them no, but I should have said, "Listening and supporting the waves of good and bad days are the best things a family can do for a CRPS/Lyme patient." Active listening and allowing a person to vent without interruption or judgment can really be uplifting. Another trick is to view the person separate from their predicament. A person is *not* their circumstances. They are a child of God whose soul may long to be set free. When I longed for someone to understand my issues, John would remark, "There is nothing they can do," which offered reality to him but pessimism for me.

Sarah often gave me the sweetest bits of compassion and encouragement. One afternoon in the car as we were returning home from a soccer game, she asked, "Mom, does anything hurt today?"

I answered, "It's a good day. Why?"

Then she said, "Last week you asked when you would have a day when nothing hurt. I told you it would be soon. And I found a penny today in car line." I suppose she was always monitoring my status. She wanted her mom back.

I felt the urge to educate others, although I still had lots to learn myself. I pleaded for my parents and family members to read more, ask questions, and gain understanding about Lyme disease. My dad retorted with, "John doesn't understand. And I know your kids don't understand. All I know is *somebody ought to do something!*" My dad didn't like to read. His preferred method of learning was speaking with others. He spoke with his uncle's friend, who used a much more expensive Rife machine from Australia. My dad then gave me the man's phone number. When I spoke with him, I realized using his Rife machine didn't cure him, but it aided him and his family members. His son seemed to benefit the most, so I spoke with him, and he noted changing his diet had been crucial.

In terms of communicating with my parents, I enjoyed simple, short phone calls from them because hardly anyone else called. When I was asleep during the day and John was home, he often answered texts on my phone in a timely manner to friends and family members. No one knew that he was the one answering the texts on my phone. It was very helpful when carpool plans needed altering or when someone needed an immediate answer.

One day, I'd been awake during the early morning hours, tossing and turning with the electrifying pain currents that I'd hoped were behind me. The pain made me want to jump off a cliff or out of my skin, as I prayed the Rosary, seeking comfort and filling my thoughts with Mother Mary holding me steady. In our dark, quiet bedroom, I lay there, shaking side to side, wondering what triggered this reaction. It was supposed to be a joyful evening. It was our twenty-first wedding anniversary. I hadn't been in a celebratory mood, but for John's sake, I made an effort to go to dinner for a gluten-free steak, salad (hold the dressing), spring water, and no yummy restaurant warm bread or complimentary anniversary dessert.

I tried to tolerate the jovial, carefree and loud customers around us, but all I wanted was to go home and get into my pajamas and under the covers so I could escape into the merriment of the Hallmark Channel. I did appreciate the beautiful flowers that John brought home before dinner, as it was a time for remembering how much I loved and cherished my husband. But then and there in that bed, I pleaded for someone to "Make it stop!" and I regretted telling Evan the same thing two days earlier.

In a dream, I kept finding pennies on the walking path, but then realized John had laid them out for me to find. I think he wanted me to be well more than anyone. He wanted to put a rush order on my healing. He wanted me to find peace and for his incessant worry to cease. He wanted things to return to normal. In reality, our time together was different. Our dates and anniversary celebrations were different. We learned to embrace simple pleasures. We went to a movie theater where I could sit in the dark with my earplugs and sometimes sunglasses, or we watched a movie in bed at home. We swam in the backyard pool, went for a walk, or dined at home on the fine china we'd received as wedding gifts. I'd have one of the meals Amber made, which were safe for me to eat, and he would pick up dinner for himself and the kids. We lit our own candles. We postponed our celebrations as needed and became grateful for the little things.

Our holiday traditions had to evolve for me as well. I no longer had gumbo for Christmas Eve and traded other holiday dishes for something I could eat. One Christmas, we went skiing. It was a minor miracle when I skied for two hours during that week away. Relaxing vacations were the best, so we usually went to the beach. Everyone was happy and occupied there, and I had a bedroom I could retreat to anytime I needed it. One afternoon, I brought a floating raft out to the beach near the seashore, plopped down on it, covered myself with a beach towel, and slept outside to the lulling of the rolling waves. We also allowed our children to bring friends along, to enhance their fun and excitement and give me more resting time.

During a private sunset conversation sitting near the seashore, John mentioned, "It's been a nice week being away from the demands of the office. I'm so relaxed here."

I was happy for him, but reminded him, "I don't ever get to leave Lyme disease behind." It was always there, lurking.

Birthdays looked different too without the traditional birthday cake. A few times, I enjoyed a store-bought gluten-free cupcake. But over the years, I preferred a homemade, healthy baked good or smoothie bowl and a candle as my celebration treat. One adventurous birthday led John and me to the local tennis courts, where we hit a few balls. My strokes weren't pretty, but it was fun! I wondered if I ever would be able to play competitive tennis again or even complete a tennis match. Health was my birthday wish each year.

Natalie, my faithful firecracker problem-solving friend, invited me to join her book club meeting. They had an entire day planned, starting with a trip into the city to a museum and dinner afterward, ending with a book discussion at her home. I told her I'd come for a short time after their fun day. When I arrived, I thought they would've been finished discussing the book, but they were in the middle of a passionate overview of its theme and characters. Then their conversations tilted to everything else going on in their lives—their next trip, jobs, involvement in their children's activities, the next book they'd gather to discuss. At the end, one friend asked if I was ready to join their book club, telling me how fun it was.

I didn't know how to answer her, so I just replied, "You all are fun." It would've been a luxury to get lost in fiction with them, but all I read were Lyme disease-related books when

I felt alright and could focus. I left there feeling hollow, yet again reminded that it was easier not to talk to normal people very often.

As my health declined, we only committed to hosting our children's friends on occasion and some Christian youth group gatherings. During those gatherings, we provided space for Jesus's life to be shared in a fun and unique way and for the youth to learn about the gospels. Basically, we provided the home, and often the food and snacks, then the leaders would take over, so there was little pressure on me. Filling our home with the teens and younger kids brought our home back to life. In addition, I was in my safe place and able to retreat as needed. Hosting adults was usually risky, on the other hand. One year, I was so grateful to be able to vacuum and get the house ready for John's office Christmas party. The party was lovely, and I was safe at home, able to escape to my bedroom as needed.

There were also times when I hated to say no. Patrick approached me, asking, "Mom, do you think we can host my group's homecoming after-party this year?"

My first answer was an enthusiastic, "Of course!" I told him we could have Sarah spend the night with a friend. I went on and on about potential plans. Patrick stopped me though, and said, "Mom, I'm more concerned about you, not Sarah."

He was right. My days were not predictable, and I knew I couldn't stay awake until 2:00 A.M., much less tolerate the noise made throughout the night. I hoped the following year it would've been another story, yet I had to cancel the T-shirt swap pizza party for Evan's homecoming group. The mom who organized their homecoming activities quickly found another home for the celebration while I lay in bed with a migraine. I was learning to surrender.

It had been eighteen months since my Lyme disease diagnosis when John planned a weekend visit with his high school friends. He did plan it to be held in our hometown in case I needed him. We were both ready for a break, and I was happy for him to have a weekend off. I prepared by having an extra sauna session during the week to alleviate my need for him. What I didn't plan on, however, were my intense suicidal thoughts following that extra sauna session. They came out of nowhere, and I didn't understand them until two days later.

I felt like I was internally about to come unglued, and I wasn't thinking straight. I was so alone and very sad. Everyone was at the high school football game, but it was yet another Friday evening at home for me, lying in bed again and watching back-to-back episodes of TLC's *Say Yes to the Dress*. I was so angry I didn't recognize myself. I didn't want to be in pain anymore. I felt disposable and that I was a burden. My family had gotten used to my "normal," but I hadn't. I longed for a better quality of life, but I was losing ground and not sure I could maintain my fight anymore. I didn't want to do it anymore. All these feelings and emotions escalated and compounded at once.

That night, I was trying to wind down and go to sleep to soothe my flailing emotions. All three kids came home later than expected. Sarah liked to be tucked in bed, but my legs plainly were not making it up the stairs. She asked Patrick to tuck her in since John was out, but Patrick was fiddling with his computer past midnight, trying to retrieve the required form for his SAT college test he was taking the following morning.

Evan called the house phone at 11:40 P.M., asking if he could spend the night at a friend's house. I had already turned my cellphone off, depending on him to be quietly dropped off at home as planned.

All the late-night chaos threw me into a tailspin. I was even more furious by this point and was so worked up that I couldn't sleep. My body reacted to it, and I felt as if I was sizzling all over. I experienced another night of deeply penetrating and burning pains beyond measure, causing me to writhe in pain hour after hour. There was absolutely no escape. My nervous system was practically ringing out, "Beware! Danger!"

The following morning, I brought Sarah to her soccer game. I was numb, angry, and still having residual suicidal thoughts, now caused by the overnight torment. John's parents met us at the soccer field. I had no words—I was so beyond exhausted and still carrying the internal rage that I had no control over. I had no more energy to even communicate with them. They must have contacted John because he called me.

"How are y'all doing?" he asked. "Do you need me to come muscle-test you?"

That was the last thing I wanted, yet the only thing that could possibly help.

"I'm sorry, but I do need you for a few minutes." He came home to muscle-test which supplements and Rife frequencies would be best for me prior to rejoining his friends for the concert and night out.

The next morning, he came home early, walking in through the kitchen door. I was still in my pajamas and baking cinnamon rolls for the kids. Sarah was half awake in front of the TV upstairs in the game room, and the boys were still asleep. The coast was clear.

Do I tell John what happened to me Friday? I contemplated. He has always been a good listener and has always worked long days. When the boys were babies and toddlers and I was a new mom without resources or family nearby, I'd vent to John about whatever stressful event happened that day in preparation for facing the stressors of the next one. But no two days were alike, and it felt as if my stressors vanished just by voicing them into the open air. Maybe this would be the same. The quiet kitchen seemed to be as good a time as any to talk to him.

"How was the concert?" I asked.

"It was okay; the guys are doing well. It was good to see everyone," he shared as he made himself a cup of coffee. "You didn't look good yesterday."

I mustered up some courage, commenting, "It was a bad night—a really bad night." My stomach jumped in my chest as the truth was emerging. My heart surged forth, and my lips tightened.

I tried suppressing it until the heaviness launched. "I was losing it. Friday night scared me. I wanted to *end* it. I wanted it all to end, but every potential ending would be more painful. It wasn't the first time."

He didn't know what to say, and I didn't expect him to counsel me. In fact, I didn't have the ability to handle *any* of his emotions, as I was trying to hold my own. I was embarrassed that I couldn't keep it together. He was about to continue the conversation, but I cut him off.

"I can't talk about this anymore." I couldn't look him in the eye or even be around him. He knew too much, and I didn't want to be judged or pitied. I walked outside on the patio to be alone with my thoughts. I knew I had dropped a bomb in the kitchen, and I had to flee.

There were times when I really wanted a counselor, yet I knew a counselor wouldn't understand my symptoms or Lyme disease and would possibly patronize or hospitalize me. They'd think these pains were all in my head. "A trash case," they'd say, "maybe an unfit mother." After church that evening, I was inspired to google "suicidal thoughts and mercury." Multiple articles were found. *Perhaps the extra sauna released too much mercury?* I'd have to be careful how often I used the sauna. The truth was that the thought of leaving my children without a mother kept me from attempting suicide. But in this recurring dark place, I understood for the first time how someone could want a way out. Now I have a much better understanding of the many ways heavy metals penetrate our bodies, including our brains, and short-circuit normal electrical nerve impulses, leaving us subject to anxiety, depression, memory loss, emotional upheaval, and migraines.

I had become very good at keeping up with appearances, although the darkness loomed in my presence. I was constantly seeking light and thankful I had my children to keep me occupied. My devotional book, *Jesus Calling*, became my lifeline as we carried onward. After the second year on his protocols, I visited Dr. Mabrey a third time. He used all the same testing methods but only added another supplement (John saw it coming) and made minor changes.

Upon my fourth visit with Dr. Mabrey and the third year on his protocols, he proclaimed, "I don't know why you aren't better yet!"

There it was. Our hope was gone in *one sentence*. After three years of following his suggestions, that's all he had to say! What were we supposed to do with that?

We went home dumbfounded. John and I couldn't believe we had dedicated ourselves *every day for three years* to this protocol and the Rife machine and had gotten *nowhere*.

"Sit quietly with Me, letting all your fears and worries bubble up to the surface of your consciousness. However, some fears surface over and over again, especially fear of the future," Sarah Young wrote for the November 9 devotional in *Jesus Calling*.

My fear of the future had reached an all-time high. I didn't know what else to do to heal, but my faith guaranteed me peace in His presence and strength to cope with whatever lay ahead. I was definitely on a "Desert Road" just like the song by Casting Crowns, filled with uncertainty of what was coming yet dependent on faith to see myself through. During the night when the pain woke me up, I kept singing another song by Casting Crowns, "Just Be Held," as my mantra to a better life. My brother once asked me if I was going to have *this* forever. The truth is, I didn't know. However, the reality of the life I once knew was indeed totally gone. I remained focused on things I could do instead of what I couldn't. If I was forced to surrender to the bed, I could help the kids study for a test, read to Sarah, or edit an English paper while lying down. The five of us reported if we'd luckily found a penny on any given day. We were constantly seeking inspiration.

Rachel Platten's "Fight Song" was very popular then. She has said that she was at a low point when she wrote the song.

I needed to remind myself to keep going—that I still believed in myself and had fight left. I adopted her song as my second theme song. I called my local Texas Lyme Disease contact. She mentioned a female doctor, located about a three-hour drive away, whom many people were seeing and liking. John drove me to an appointment. The ride itself was very difficult, dragging on as if it was a three-day drive instead of three hours. The doctor, who was very compassionate, suggested new and different supplements, foods for chronic fatigue, IV vitamin C, and juicing for better detoxing. I tried some of the supplements she suggested, but they only made me feel worse. I dismissed her advice. I didn't understand juicing and was uncertain of IV vitamin C.

My sweet neighbor listened to talk radio often. She had heard about a lady treating her Lyme disease with bee venom therapy (BVT). She told me about it and encouraged me to never give up. When you are willing to sting yourself with live bees in order to heal, you are without a doubt at rock bottom!

We found an online farm that actually mailed us *live* bees in a box, along with special tweezers. Before we began my BVT, I purchased an EpiPen for $436.02 to have on hand just in case I needed it. People were complaining about the pharmaceutical cost of the EpiPens then and arguing about coverage with their insurance companies. John used the special tweezers to gather each bee and then placed the stinger on my back, per the included instructions from the farm. Yes, it hurt, but not hardly as much as the burning I experienced in my body. The bee venom acted like a steroid and gave me the energy to get out of the house and get things done. The following day, however, I would usually crash. It was a cycle, and I had gotten used to it.

Sometimes, a bee would escape from the small wooden bee box we set on the counter. It would fly all around our large bathroom, into the shower, above the bathtub, around the chandelier, back and forth to the mirrored wall. John would be chasing it down frantically, jumping on the bathtub ledge, climbing into the shower. "Watch out!" he'd scream, pushing me aside to save us from the inch-long buzzing bee. "Close the doors," he'd yell, giving the little guy limited flight path parameters. I sat still and watched with laughter on the inside, knowing I was going to get stung anyway.

I joined a BVT Facebook group and read stories of how some people felt better while others felt worse. When we traveled to the beach in Alabama that summer, I googled the state beekeeping association and made some calls until I found a man willing to give me twelve bees. He laughed out loud and said I would need a lot more than twelve bees to make honey. I explained BVT to him, and he agreed to meet me in the YMCA parking lot for our bee exchange. We continued BVT for eight months, until my mother's friend had another idea.

CHAPTER 8

Something New

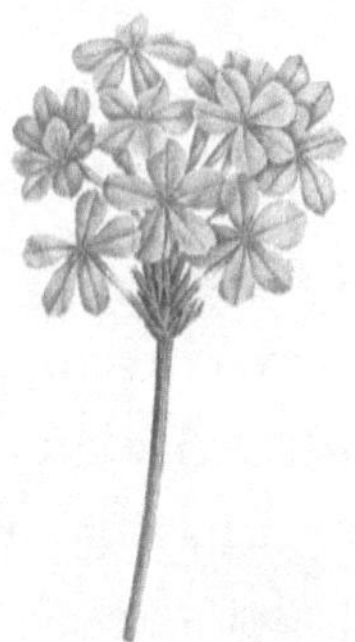

"Hı Moм," I answered the phone.

"Hi Deb. Are you feeling okay today? I have some news for you. I just spoke with Nancy (her older prayer-group friend), and she has some new information about Lyme disease."

"What could Nancy possibly know about Lyme?"

"She was visiting her sister over the Christmas holidays, and she told her about you and how you've been struggling. Her sister then told her about a new book with a different take on Lyme disease. Nancy said that tick bites aren't the cause of Lyme disease and mentioned the author has been given a healing gift. At age four, he was able to tell his grandmother she had lung cancer!"

"At age four, he told his grandmother she had lung cancer?"

"That's what she said, Deb. Maybe you should get the book?"

"I don't know, Mom. I've already read all I could find about Lyme disease. I've never come across anything like what you're talking about. There are lots of people who take advantage of Lyme patients, so I'm not sure."

"How about you get the book and read it for your own discernment? I'll text you the title. I hope it will help you, honey!"

At first, I assumed it was just another Lyme book full of broken promises. But my mom had caught my attention when she related the author's story of being only four years old and telling his grandmother she had lung cancer. So, I ordered the book *Medical Medium: Secrets Behind Chronic and Mystery Illness and How to Finally Heal* by Anthony William. His shocking outburst at a family dinner had prompted his grandmother to seek medical attention, and sure enough, she was diagnosed with lung cancer following an X-ray.

The other part of the conversation with my mom, which had also caught my attention, was how Nancy relayed the message of Lyme disease *not* being transmitted by ticks. It was profoundly different and new information! When the book arrived at my doorstep, I went straight to the chapter on Lyme disease.

William begins the chapter with a warning about Lyme disease, where he tells the readers to be aware of the "Lyme trap." He then states that the greatest mistake of modern medical history is the belief that Lyme disease is caused by the bacterium, *Borrelia burgdorferi. What? What does he mean?* Everyone believes *Borrelia burgdorferi* is the cause of Lyme disease, as stated in the Lyme literature.

Why is this belief a *trap*? William explains the current treatment for Lyme disease is to prescribe antibiotics to treat the bacteria, but that the *Borrelia burgdorferi* bacterium is actually *harmless and is carried by every animal and human being on the planet, posing no health risk at all!* In addition, he claims the problem with the antibiotics is two-fold. The harsh antibiotics bruise already sensitive nerves. Patients are taught that the antibiotics will cause a beneficial Jarisch-Herxheimer reaction (or bacterial die-off as the body detoxes). However, William insists that the reaction is actually a step in the *wrong* direction—it's a problem, a red flag, a lack of progress. On top of that, he adds the antibiotics used to treat Lyme disease actually make the real culprit grow bigger and stronger, sabotaging any chance of a cure. Sounded like a trap to me, and I'd already fallen for it.

I didn't take the antibiotics, yet I took loads of antimicrobial supplements that produced excruciating nerve pain daily. I had been taught it was the only way to heal Lyme disease. I thought it was a better way to heal than by ingesting antibiotics. I had no idea that I was harming myself on my quest to heal.

William says the true cause of Lyme disease is a variety of viruses in the herpes family, and that the disease varies in each individual because there are numerous strains of each virus. He points to the Epstein-Barr virus (EBV), also known as human herpesvirus 4 (HHV-4), stating there are over sixty varieties; however, only *one* variety is known and recognized by modern medicine. In addition to over sixty EBV varieties, he states the other herpetic viruses contributing to Lyme disease symptoms are the multiple varieties of shingles (over thirty), HHV-6 (over twenty), HHV-7, herpes simplex (two), and cytomegalovirus (CMV, twenty), although only one type is currently known for most of them. That leaves roughly 133+ viruses possibly unaccounted for and unable to be tested. These viruses could be part of the missing link, contributing to the confusion over people suffering from numerous mysterious symptoms.

In his SoundCloud podcast, "Truth About Multiple Sclerosis," William states that more and more people who have or would have received an MS diagnosis are now being funneled into a Lyme disease diagnosis. He explains when Lyme disease was first recognized in the 1970s, there were no antiviral pharmaceuticals available to treat viruses, but there were steroids and antibiotics available to treat bacterial infections. William says almost 85% of Lyme patients grow worse with antibiotic treatment for their viral condition, and 15% of them show improvement when they add beneficial alternate treatments such as IV vitamin C and supplements like cat's claw.

Lyme disease is known as "the great imitator" of over three hundred symptoms. It's no wonder the current poor Lyme testing methods aren't reliable. The testing methods have been poor from the start, but for some reason, they are still being utilized today. How can the current testing methods be accurate if we aren't testing for the correct pathogens up front? William points to many viruses as the cause of the disease—viruses that are elusive to our doctors and healthcare workers because they are undiscovered, unnamed, and don't show up on blood tests. This is a problem! Yet, the concept was enlightening to me. It makes so much sense that viruses could be to blame because they cause nerve issues and bacteria do not. If the cause is viral, antibiotics then wouldn't work because they don't kill viruses—they kill bacteria.

In his book, Anthony William explains how streptococcus bacteria is the best friend of EBV, most often found together. Those Lyme patients who reported feeling better on antibiotics probably felt better due to a lower strep bacteria count instead of a lower viral count; they could've experienced the virus going dormant or used additional alternate treatments that did the trick. A viral cause would explain Lyme patients relapsing or never healing with long-term antibiotics. But what about those Lyme patients who had a bull's-eye rash and healed after two weeks of antibiotics? William says the rash is the body fighting a normal bacterial staph infection from a spider bite, bee sting, or tick bite, all of which leave part of the creature lodged in your skin. What a logical explanation for the rash! The author then declares, "For the record, *Borrelia* has never been found and cultured from a bull's-eye, nor has *Babesia* or *Bartonella*." How in the world has this simplicity eluded us for over fifty years since Lyme was first studied in 1975? Oh, that's right, it was thought to be a *viral cause* in the first place!

Why has the confusion over Lyme disease continued for over fifty years? Why hasn't anything changed? According to scientific journalist and author Pamela Weintraub, when there was an investigation into expanding the Lyme definition from an acute infection to a chronic infection, the Connecticut attorney general found the author's conflicts of the Infectious Diseases Society of America (IDSA) Lyme disease guideline to be profound:

They consulted for big Pharma and owned Lyme-related patents; they received fees as expert witnesses in medical-malpractice, civil, and criminal cases related to Lyme disease;

and they were paid by insurance companies to field—and help reject—Lyme-related claims. Of the fourteen authors, nine received money from vaccine manufacturers and four were funded to create test kits, products that would be more likely to reap profit if the definition of Lyme disease remained essentially unchanged.

Where there is confusion, there is profit. If they didn't want to expand the definition of Lyme disease from an acute bacterial infection to a chronic bacterial infection, there was no way a viral cause would be exposed now. On July 12, 2013, CNN published an article by Pamela Weintraub titled, "Why You Should Be Afraid of Lyme Disease." In it, she wrote of her family's struggles with Lyme disease and warned the public that those in power were downplaying the disease, stating, "The real science deniers are those circling the wagons around outdated studies, leaving patients desperate and sick while protecting their academic turf."

The following day, Lorraine Johnson (then CEO of lymedisease.org) promoted Pam's article in her Lyme Policy Wonk blog, explaining there was a small group of researchers who had a lock on research funding for Lyme disease. She credited Mary Beth Pfeiffer at the *Poughkeepsie Journal* for exposing a broken peer review due to the CDC and NIH working with the IDSA to cancel legislation for fair research. Johnson wrote:

> Science depends on the free marketplace of ideas. Few scientists refute their own theories; their rivals do. What happens when researchers supporting one paradigm "get hold of some institutional position of power (a scientific journal, a research institute) and impose their favorite 'line' of research there, lead-

ing to a dead end." If you can successfully exclude your rivals, you have the whole playing field to yourself. But what is produced is dead-end science that does not improve patient care.

Hopefully, one day science will fully prevail. There are already studies starting to link EBV to MS, lupus, and some cancers. However, clearly there has been a conflict of interest in all things Lyme-related since it was first investigated in Lyme, Connecticut. Perhaps Anthony William is onto something— something new!

I realized it was time for me to do my own research. So, I visited my primary care provider and asked for an EBV test. Previous testing of all sorts proved unhelpful, so I didn't have high expectations. A week later, I slowly drove to the nearby office for my results. In a frigid waiting room, I sat between children's toys and a table full of magazines, waiting and wondering what the results would show. Slumped over with my head resting in my hand, I thought about how there are potentially over sixty varieties of the EBV virus. The chances of my having the one EBV virus strain that the medical field tests for were slim.

A red-headed nurse called my name, interrupting my thoughts. She escorted me to a room with disposable paper newly draped over the exam table. After my vital signs showed within normal limits, the nurse asked, "What is your preferred pharmacy?"

It's always the first question. The Southern belle in me has often thought the first question should be: *How are you today?* When all the obligatory questions were out of the way, I was left alone to think about my next moves, crossing my fingers as

I hoped for direction. In walked an older doctor with glasses on his face and cotton-ball hair in clumps above his ears.

"Hello, your EBV test has a result of 103."

I remained calm, but in my head, I was completely blown away. My EBV blood test was *off the charts!* The normal range is 0.0–17.9, and the positive result is greater than 21.9. Did the positive EBV test explain the chronic fatigue and flu-like aches, just as William said?

The buttoned-up and well-dressed doctor had instructions. "It's best to get plenty of rest, avoid strenuous activity, hydrate, and use over-the-counter medications as needed."

That's it? I asked for more. "I've been having these symptoms for almost five years. Do you have any other suggestions?"

He looked at me with compassion in his eyes, gave me a tender pat on the back, and said, "You take good care, and let me know if I can do anything for you." Before I knew it, another white coat had walked away from me and left the room.

I thought this was going to be the first test of any kind bearing a revelation. *Was it finally an honest answer and a true diagnosis?* I finally felt validated and ready to act, as my new book would provide a way to heal, giving me steps back to health. I didn't have another option. All my other options were exhausted.

John, a natural-born critic, particularly perked up. He felt that he finally had a concrete medical explanation for my lack of life. He felt he had something concrete to tell our family and friends: "Deborah has the Epstein-Barr virus." He, too, believed my blood test was validating.

But mostly our family and friends were stuck on my Lyme disease diagnosis, had long forgotten about my CRPS diagnosis, and were skeptical of any new diagnoses. I still kept receiving questions. "So, do you have Lyme disease?" they would ask. "That's a can of worms," I'd reply. "Yes, I have Lyme disease symptoms; however, modern medicine dictates the cause of Lyme is bacterial, and the new information I have spells out the cause as the Epstein-Barr virus and other assorted undiscovered viruses." This was (and still is) very confusing to the masses. It's simply not black-and-white. Most people have a need to believe in modern science and that medicine won't fail them and will keep them safe. But modern science and medicine have both failed me, along with others, struggling with chronic illness. It was time for something new.

It is widely known that the Epstein-Barr virus has infected over ninety percent of the global population. William writes EBV is easily contractible from your parents as a baby at birth, during blood transfusions, and via the exchange of bodily fluids. I'd had a complete emergency blood transfer at birth due to complications of an Rh incompatibility. Keep in mind that because most viruses are undiscovered, they aren't filtered from donated blood. Is it possible to have this virus and not even know it? Most of us do. Because it's so widespread, doctors don't get alarmed at elevated blood test results. My friend, Dr. Phan, led me to the EBV Global Institute site. There I learned the specific EBV blood test that I was given—the VCA IgG—remains elevated for life and alone doesn't deem a chronic EBV condition. However, a very high result could raise a red flag. My flag was highly raised to attention as I learned about the elusive EBV virus.

In his book, William expands on four stages of the Epstein-Barr virus. He says in Stage One, EBV is dormant in your bloodstream, is undetectable through tests, and causes no symptoms. In Stage Two, EBV challenges your immune system, presenting itself as mononucleosis (mono for short), which is common among teens and young adults, contagious, and detectable with a blood test. It's the EBV we are familiar with—Stage Two.

William calls out the sneaky virus, as it seeks a long-term home in the liver, spleen, and/or reproductive organs, eating poisons that accumulate in these organs and then nesting there in Stage Three. In Stage Three, he explains, EBV is quite patient. It can lie dormant for years, become problematic by burrowing deeper into the organs, or become apparent when the immune system is weakened. It then travels to the thyroid, all while the viral load increases in numbers. Yet a blood test will only indicate a past infection at that point. The thyroid, however, takes the hit, erupting in all types of thyroid issues, leaving the cause unknown to health professionals and patients alike. William boldly announces that it's in this stage when the viral cells can "get caught" traveling via the bloodstream from the liver to the thyroid. They then can be found in lymph nodes and tissue surrounding the breasts, being a major part of an unknown breast cancer cause.

William believes it's Stage Four where the EBV reaches its goal of inflaming the central nervous system (the main issue of Lyme disease), causing several strange symptoms, like heart palpitations, migrating aches and pains, numbness and tingling, mysterious fatigue, and unexplainable nerve pain. Patients suffering are out of luck when this happens, because blood tests, X-rays, and scans usually won't reveal the problem. As a result, doctors won't realize the EBV is inflaming the nerves. William sums it up by stating, "Stage Four Epstein-Barr is therefore a major source of mystery illness—that is, neurological problems that cause doctors massive confusion." And even if a blood test identifies the EBV as a problem, it won't be linked to a neurological problem, leaving patients hopping from doctor to doctor, seeking answers. Sounds familiar, right? I believe this was the beginning of when I finally began to understand my issues.

Remember, my journey began with an immobile hand following a fractured wrist and the CRPS label of unexplained severe pain. William expanded my understanding of Stage Four EBV:

> When the nerve is injured, the root hairs pop off the sides of the nerve sheath. EBV looks for those openings and grabs on to them. If it succeeds, it can keep the area inflamed for years. As a result, you can have a relatively small injury that remains flared up and causes you continual pain.

This is exactly what happened to me! I broke my wrist; it became inflamed, along with the rest of my body, and caused continual pain even after the fracture fully healed. *This guy is a genius!* He adds, in Stage Four, neurological symptoms can also occur without an injury because some EBV varieties produce neurotoxins that inflame the nerves, resulting in "muscle pain, joint pain, painful tender points, back pain, tingling and/or numbness in the hands and feet, jerking and spasms, tinnitus (ringing, buzzing, humming, or popping sounds in the ears), migraines, ongoing fatigue, dizziness, eye floaters, insomnia, unrestful sleep, and night sweats." He was capturing reasons for all my symptoms. *What else did he know?*

In this book, he lists the twenty-four most common Lyme disease triggers, which he says trigger the herpes virus already in our bodies, even if we are unaware. Several of these triggers pertained to my history: the removal of mercury-based dental amalgam fillings; mercury ingestion from frequently eating seafood; being around and consuming pesticides, herbicides, and fungicides; a history of insecticide usage in the home; a history of having the flu; bee stings; overprescribed medications (i.e., antibiotics as a kid for chronic sinusitis); physical injuries; and fresh paint. He adds, "There's roughly a 75 percent chance that one or more of the above triggers occurred within three months to a year of the onset of your symptoms." He was on point, as we had previously moved into a freshly painted home six months prior to my injury, and my symptoms had evolved following the triggering wrist injury. Surprisingly, a tick bite is the *least common trigger* on his list.

He knew even more. He explained the itching, burning, and stabbing pain were from a shingles virus, but not the one we recognize today as a red rash and pustules. He dedicates an entire chapter to the shingles virus, writing there are thirty-one varieties but addresses the most common fifteen types: seven of which produce rashes and eight of which don't. According to William, the shingles viruses without rashes have the potential to cause *even more* internal pain and nerve injury than the strains that cause rashes. The strains matching my symptoms were the non-rash kind—the "maddening itch shingles," the "frozen shoulder shingles," the "arm and leg burning shingles," the "neuralgic shingles," and the "body on fire shingles," referencing the burning pain of CRPS.

Next, he shed light on the foods I'd been avoiding as nightshades. In book two of his series, *Medical Medium Life-Changing Foods, Expanded Edition*, he writes about nightshade fear, clearing up the misconception that potatoes, tomatoes, peppers, and eggplants aggravate conditions like arthritis. He points to the real nightshade issues: the poisonous dark nightshade berries found in the woods, and also eating anything at an unripe stage. He states,

> Most green bell peppers that you'll see on the grocery store shelf are just unripe versions of the red bell peppers nearby. Opt for the red ones, because a green pepper or tomato (unless it's a variety that's green when ripe) is still in the nightshade realm and can be an irritant. (*Anything* at such an unripe stage can be irritating.) Once ripe, the fruit itself is no longer actually a nightshade.

Suddenly, I realized my over-the-top added layer of pain from the food items I had ingested was a result of eating unripe fruits. The restaurant had told me their green beans were marinated in green peppers, and I safely assume that the peppers in the guacamole I bought were unripe as well. This information gave me more food options to add to my diet. To this day, I still don't eat green bell peppers.

What's interesting is I grew up on the "holy trinity" of Cajun cooking—onions, bell peppers, and celery as a base for crawfish etouffee, gumbo, and jambalaya. I know most of the time that green bell peppers were used in cooking when I was younger, and they didn't bother me at all. But at this point in my life, the once-dormant viruses were wreaking havoc and inflaming me from the inside out. So, the true unripe nightshades needed to be avoided without fail.

I was essentially "reading for a better life," and I seemingly was finding it. Missing pieces of the puzzle were falling into place, creating a picture of hope where there once was despair. William gave me an explanation of what was *truly* physiologically happening inside of me and releasing the accusation from others of something being psychologically wrong with me. He silently spoke to me:

> Your EBV-related health problems aren't the result of anything you did wrong or any moral failing. You didn't make this happen, and you're in no way to blame. You did not manifest this; you did not attract this. You're a vibrant, wonderful human being and you have every God-given right to heal. You *deserve* to heal.

No one else has been able to come up with such profound and vivid explanations. He even acknowledged the few things that made me feel good, highlighting how the infrared sauna and massage as tolerated were beneficial detox methods. I was all in, but my family was not.

William is *not* a doctor, although he holds great respect for doctors and healthcare workers and says he helps them with their most difficult cases. He says he works for God. He doesn't claim to have honed this information on his own. He has been guided by God's Spirit of Compassion (SOC)—a voice he hears outside of his ear, giving him advanced healing information beyond the current scope of both traditional and alternative medical communities. It was this voice who told him about his grandmother's lung cancer. It was this voice that taught William about the healing properties of the produce in his great-grandpa's garden in Italy. In the *Medical Medium Podcast* episode titled "A Chat with My Dad Part 3," William and his father reminisce about how his great-grandparents knew he was gifted, yet they wanted to protect him from a cruel world because he was so young. They revealed it was his great-grandfather who first coined him as the "little medical medium."

William's story is absolutely incredible, and a must-read included at the beginning of his first book. He shares his struggle to accept this gift for humanity and the sacrifice he's made to live such a unique life with a massive responsibility. He humbly offers he has helped tens of thousands of people fully recover from their ailments and taught them how to maintain a vibrant life. He credits working for God with the Spirit of Compassion. He remarks,

> This book unveils many of Spirit's most precious medical secrets. It's the answer for anyone who's suffering from a chronic condition or a mystery illness that doctors haven't been able to resolve. It's not just a book for people who are sick, though. It's a book for every person on the planet.

He closes Chapter 1 explaining no other medium alive does what he does—works as a messenger to provide clear and advanced health information from a spirit voice.

Christianity and the Bible warn of the evildoings of mediums. But this man states he works for God, and no evil can be found on the pages of his books. In fact, what is found amid the information is the opposite of evil. There is truth, hope, and understanding. There are answers to all my questions and all the mysterious symptoms I have experienced. There is a miracle! It has been said our God works in mysterious ways! Proverbs 16:16 states, "How much better to acquire wisdom than gold! To acquire understanding is more desirable than silver."

I had uncovered the most significant information yet, but no one in my family seemed to be on board. John was completely checked out. We had been burned so badly from so many previous attempts at healing. He was angry and distant, and he had given up on ever finding a cure. He had surrendered to the notion of never having a healthy wife.

"John, please read the book. I think you'll understand why I'm doing this," I pleaded. Yet, he never picked it up.

Bids came in to purchase John's company, and since we were no longer muscle-testing supplements, we were no longer tethered to working on that task. I was flying solo. I wished John had been supportive of my new attempt at healing. However, he was stumped by the idea of a medium, and he wasn't the only one in the family who felt this way.

The kids were doing their own things. Hospitable and adventurous Patrick brought friends home from college to and from Florida for their spring break. Sarah had turned thirteen and surprised herself as she came in first place at her junior high district track meet in the 100 hurdles, the 4×200 relay, and the 4×100 relay. (Both of her relays broke the school records.) Athletic and on-the-go Evan had to slow down due to ankle surgery and would be on crutches for a month. Both of our parents were in town supporting their grandkids. They didn't understand my new protocol. They didn't ask many questions either, and when they did, they asked John, as if I weren't of sound mind or body. I think everyone still believed a medical doctor was the answer. They didn't understand traditional medicine could not help me, which made me feel even more alienated.

My charismatic dad avoided me during one visit. One morning, I joined him in the kitchen where he was working on his crossword puzzle. He and John were similar in many ways; they were both heavy thinkers. He was drinking his coffee with milk and sweetener, and I was sipping on my lemon honey water.

"Deb, are you sure about this new protocol?"

"I have some validating information from the book, explaining all the issues I have been having for so long."

"I don't know about using a protocol from a medium, Deb? That's just not how I think," he blurted out. "How confident are you in this new plan?"

Had he forgotten the element of the experimental in my health case? "I know this is weird, Dad. My entire journey has been weird!" I was over it being weird and just desperately wanted to heal. I couldn't think of a better way to receive healing than from the divine—a pure source without an agenda.

So, to answer my dad's question, I simply said, "I think these protocols may help my case. The explanations add up, and it makes sense physiologically." My protective dad had nothing else to say. He was cautious but didn't know enough to refute this decision. I carried onward and hoped I would see *The Way* when they didn't. I hoped the Medical Medium information filled in the missing pieces that they didn't know were missing.

CHAPTER 9

It's a Process

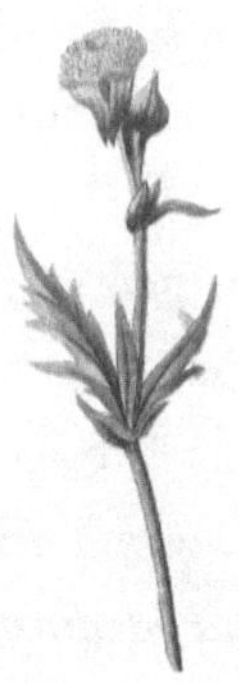

HAVE YOU HEARD THE parable of the drowning man? It's
a non-biblical story used worldwide in religious ceremonies and
even in the workplace. It begins with a man stuck in his home as
flood waters were rising. He knew with all his might the Lord
God would come and save him because he was devoutly faithful.

His neighbor drove by in a pickup truck, offering him a ride
to safety. "No thanks," the man calls out. "God will save me!"
So, the neighbor drove away.

Soon, the man had to climb onto his rooftop, as the water
had submerged his entire home. A motorboat cruised up to the
man's home, and the boat's captain offered the man a spot on
the boat. "I don't need a spot; I'm waiting for God to come," he
called out, resulting in the boat propelling away.

An hour later, an emergency rescue helicopter flew over, patrolling the area. They dropped a ladder down to the man and instructed him to climb up the ladder into the helicopter. The man refused, declaring, "God will be here any minute to save me." So, the helicopter flew away.

Sadly, the man drowned. When he got to heaven, he furiously demanded answers for God's absence during his time of need.

"I sent you a pickup truck, a motorboat, and an emergency rescue helicopter. What more could you have needed?" God inquired.

God has always used his people to help each other, in biblical times and still today. He instructs us with the Golden Rule to treat others as we would like to be treated. Figuratively, I was that man on the roof, about to drown, until I found the answers in the book *Medical Medium* by Anthony William and the Spirit of Compassion. Despite my family's disapproval, I grabbed onto the Medical Medium's messages with both hands as my life preserver. After years of suffering and confusion, Medical Medium answered ten fundamental questions that were the foundation of my healing journey.

1. Why do we get sick?

William titles the following Unforgiving Six as the most serious and merciless health threats of the present day and the true cause of chronic and mystery illness. We are always wondering *why* we get sick. William's two *Life-Changing Foods* books are the only place to receive the truth to that question! We become frustrated with our friends and family members who just can't get it together, become forgetful, have strange behavior, or fly off the handle. But when you understand everything that they are up against in the fight to stay healthy, perhaps you'll have more compassion for them and for yourself. The Unforgiving Six invisible factors are as follows:

1. PATHOGENIC EXPLOSION: Including viral explosion (described further in Chapter 8), bacterial riptides, destructive fungi, superbugs, and intestinal parasites.

2. APPLICATIONS: Dichlorodiphenyltrichloroethane, also known as DDT, is an insecticide known to be one of the most toxic chemicals ever created. Although outlawed in the United States in 1972, it is still being used in some countries. Over thirty other applications fall into this category alongside DDT, including popular chemicals used every day. Such items are listed in William's latest *Life-Changing Foods* book.

3. RADIATION: Including atmospheric fallout from catastrophic events like Hiroshima's atomic bomb, the Chernobyl and Fukushima nuclear disasters, current nuclear weapon and nuclear plant exposure, medical tests (e.g., CT scans, PET scans, fluoroscopy, and X-rays), airplane travel, computerized devices, food and water supply contamination, and inherited exposure.

4. TOXIC HEAVY METALS: See question #6 on page 158.

5. ADRENALINE TRIGGERS: Includes triggers from

caffeine; alcohol; toxic processed food with additives, preservatives, and fillers; and a high-fat diet.

6. CIVILIZATION SABOTAGE: Includes toxic burning, such as vaping, cigarettes, and cigar smoke; trash burning; agricultural burning; industrial burning; burning of treated firewood; excessive blood draws (more information can be found in William's *Brain Saver* book); and mind control (the world is full of agendas conditioning people negatively leading to emotional eating and turning them away from God—we already know this, so be mindful).

This list might seem overwhelming, but it is meant for awareness. While some things are out of our control, there are others that we can refuse or reduce in our own environments. In *Life-Changing Foods*, William states that more than seven billion people worldwide deal with mystery illnesses. He adds that in twenty years' time, every female born will be almost guaranteed to face breast cancer unless they learn how to protect themselves. William refutes the autoimmune theory, which states real symptoms are being caused by a person's own confused immune system, viewing parts of the body as an invader and perpetually attacking itself. He, along with the SOC, says, our bodies do not attack themselves, and our genes aren't to blame. Instead, he says our bodies react to being attacked by pathogens like viruses and bacteria. In addition, our bodies carry the Unforgiving Six as inherited toxins and contaminants, and our genes aren't the problem. He lays the blame on the Unforgiving Six existing in our bodies as to why we become physically and/or mentally ill. Our bodies can be considered wonderful and perfectly made and *able to heal*!

2. How can we heal?

Using food as medicine is key to healing the Medical Medium way. So, what can we do to counteract the Unforgiving Six? William gives us what he refers to as the Holy Five:

1. FRUITS

2. LEAFY GREENS

3. VEGETABLES

4. HERBS AND SPICES

5. WILD FOODS

By ingesting these Holy Five, we can extract the Unforgiving Six from our bodies. He elaborates on over ninety foods in *Life-Changing Foods*. William describes the function of these foods, the conditions and symptoms that benefit from consuming these foods, which of the Holy Five foods remove toxins, and also the emotional support and spiritual lessons the Holy Five provide.

I had no idea that food could provide lessons for us. I thought food was just for survival. For example, avocados are described as the "mother fruit" and are considered to be the closest food on the planet to breast milk, having nurturing qualities and over twenty-five nutrients. They are instrumental in soothing the gut and restoring the central nervous system, while aiding the skin with hydration for anti-aging effects and giving the immune system a boost. Avocados can fill you up spiritually with nurturing motherly love, which you can then pass on to your loved ones.

Mangoes teach us how to handle extremely heated situations as we internalize their inner coolness. They can emotionally aid us when we feel abandoned or lonely because they hold the power of manifestation. When we eat them, they enable us to change our direction and open ourselves up to more opportunities for experiencing joy. This popular fruit is also a powerful anti-cancer food. When eaten before bed, it can act as a sleeping aid due to its combination of phytochemicals, amino acids, fructose, and glucose that restore depleted brain neurotransmitters.

Leafy greens aren't just food to cover with salad dressing. Their purpose is magnificent for our well-being. William writes leafy greens are wonderful healers of intestinal disorders over time, as they increase beneficial hydrochloric acid in the gut and create true alkalinity in our body systems. They are excellent aids for the purging of toxins from the lymphatic system and liver. Leafy greens enable us to detach and release old toxic emotions as they physically clear toxins from our bodies. William adds that spinach is a top leafy green and states his spinach soup recipe has changed lives globally, helping people rid themselves of their ailments.

One of our most beloved vegetables is the potato. Potatoes, which grow in clusters like a large family or an army of loved ones, spiritually fight for you when eaten by energetically passing along a sense of belonging to a wide familial support group. The ultimate underdog, potatoes are full of potential, offering us foundation, humble strength, and grounding wisdom to set our egos aside. Potatoes can be vital to our physical health, if ingested without the added fat and oil often associated with them. In their natural state, potatoes are our allies in the fight against chronic illness as they're filled with the amino acid lysine, a powerful weapon against cancer, liver disease, and multiple viruses. William encourages us to think twice about the misleading rumors of potatoes being an unhealthy white food, as their skins are full of color. They are truly one of the greatest gifts on Earth.

Cat's claw, an often-overlooked miracle medicinal herb from the jungle, teaches us to examine what gifts we might be bypassing in our own lives. It reveals that what we once thought was impossible is now close by and attainable, such as our very own healing. This herb contains bioactive pharma compounds, superseding traditional pharmaceuticals, in addition to antiviral, antiparasitic, and antibacterial properties. Remarkably, bacterial pathogens cannot become resistant to cat's claw like they do with synthetic antibiotics. While cat's claw is an amazing tool for most, William does point out that you should skip it if you're pregnant or trying to conceive. This herb has been strategic in my healing, as it lowered my pathogen load and continues to be a regular staple for me in tincture form.

In addition to fruits, leafy greens, vegetables, herbs, and spices, William encourages ingesting what he calls wild foods. What are they exactly? He describes them as foods that have survived extremes and are experts at thriving, helping us to adapt to what life throws at us. He believes they're the secret to a fresh start to true healing when you have been sick with a chronic illness. Wild foods can evoke even more miraculous healing powers than the others previously mentioned. For instance, *wild* blueberries are revered above all by William as the "resurrection" food—the most powerful food on the planet. He writes, "There is not a cancer that *wild* [emphasis added] blueberries cannot prevent, nor a disease known to humankind that *wild* blueberries cannot protect you from."

Atlantic sea vegetables, or seaweeds, are wild foods from the ocean, aiding in just about any illness. They absorb and deactivate the harmful frequency of heavy metals, radiation, and other toxins, and hold on to them until they exit the body together. The seaweeds relieve our bodies of poisons and leave behind over fifty health-promoting, nutritious minerals. William declares dulse seaweed as the most effective sea vegetable for removing toxic heavy metals from the body.

Finally, rose hips, which are the round fruits that develop after the flowering of certain rose plants, are also beneficial wild foods. They can be eaten or dried and then brewed up as a tea. In fact, I drank rose hips tea for my heart palpitations. According to William's *Life-Changing Foods* book, the vitamin C found in rose hips dissolves a biofilm, or sticky jelly substance, which can get caught in the heart's valves and is a hidden cause of mystery heart palpitations, tachycardia, atrial fibrillation, and arrhythmia. Where does this sticky substance come from? It's debris left over from the Epstein-Barr virus being active in the body. The biofilm is formed when the virus gives off neurotoxins and dermatoxins.

Not only do these foods work as single agents, but they also have synergistic effects, as William states in his books. As I mentioned previously, the versatile mango can be used as a sleeping aid when eaten at night. But when eaten during the day with celery sticks or greens, it can give you an energy boost. Asparagus and broccoli each have beneficial qualities, but when eaten together, broccoli actually heightens the cancer-fighting compounds found in asparagus. Cauliflower and seaweed, when eaten together, help you to detox from chlorine, harmful fluoride, and radiation, while coconut enhances the healing capabilities of anything it is paired with.

Part of healing is building your emotional and spiritual fortitude by taking in the gifts of the many living foods. I know that being able to add fully ripened potatoes and tomatoes back into my diet boosted my healing tremendously. Finding out the truth about beneficial foods took my guesswork out of avoiding harmful foods. This information isn't given as just more deception or to sell products. It's completely life-changing.

I am only scratching the surface here in listing healing foods. William describes many living foods in greater depth, not only in his books, but also on his website (medicalmedium.com), social media platforms, and podcasts. He adds that what's most remarkable about our consumption of more of the Holy Five foods is noticing how our taste buds change over time and our desire for fresh ingredients expands. I never thought I'd like brussels sprouts, but now I eat them all the time using the Medical Medium recipes. There is so much to learn given all this new information. It's crucial to our health that we view and understand these living foods for what they really are—our salvation.

3. *What foods and supplements should I avoid?*

William writes about troublemaker foods in a chapter titled "What Not to Eat" in his revised first book. This chapter also includes details of which supplements to avoid. What I like about this chapter is that he explains *why* each food and supplement should be avoided. He educates that the foods and supplements act as food for the pathogens, annoy the digestive system, or poorly affect the brain and nervous system.

Remember all the talk about *inflammation* earlier in this book? William explains when inflammation isn't from an injury, it originates from a pathogen. Furthermore, it's the result of a pathogen *feeding* on troublemaker foods and then releasing neurotoxins and dermatoxins in the process. It's the neurotoxins and dermatoxins that cause inflammation, which explains why some people have food intolerances and others do not. When that person eats a certain food, pathogens in their body feed on that food, causing toxins to be released, resulting in their discomfort. Most foods alone don't cause inflammation, with canola oil being the exception.

To heal the Medical Medium way, you are encouraged to reduce/remove the troublemaker foods and supplements from your diet and then replace them by adding more life-changing foods and supplements to aid you in your return to health and disease prevention. If you're in a pinch, search "Medical Medium Foods to Avoid for Healing Chronic Illness" online for the list of harmful foods. Know that the book, *Medical Medium Brain Saver*, expands on this list of harmful foods, supplements, and chemicals. You can also search "Medical Medium Supplements to Avoid for Healing Chronic Illness."

In hindsight, I wished I'd had this information five years prior to finding the Medical Medium book series because I had eaten many troublemaker foods along the way and taken several troublemaker supplements, making my case even worse. For example, I took over-the-counter iron supplements for anemia. The iron was acting as a metal food source for the viral pathogens in my body, which caused my anemia in the first place. William suggests using plant-based iron supplements and eating specific plant-based foods high in iron to improve anemia. I also ate and baked with eggs until I learned they are a top troublemaker food. You can find out more information about eggs by checking out William's books, social media, and two podcasts detailing *why* eggs are considered a troublemaker food. He suggests eggs be avoided by women with polycystic ovary syndrome (PCOS) and breast cancer and by anyone with a chronic illness.

4. What supplements should I take?

William emphatically and repeatedly states that eating the proper foods and eliminating troublemaker ones are our primary defense against disease. But in today's toxic world, he says most of us can benefit from some supplements to aid our body in reaching its full healthy potential, and some need supplements to fight infections.

When I began reading the Medical Medium book series in 2017, some of William's clients were teaching his information, and their contact information was listed on his website. Two of them assisted me with deciding which supplements to take. It was a bit of trial and error, in addition to painfully learning that I could hardly tolerate certain supplements. I learned to only ingest a few drops at a time when I began a new supplement. While no such contact list can be found on his website today, a plethora of information can be found there about supplementation. Other supplement information can be found on his social media and in his books. (Hint: William notes four baseline supplements to take, while Muneeza Ahmed, a client of his who also shares his information, mentions what she calls the Core Seven antiviral supplements.)

Of course, which supplements you take, along with their dosages, depends on your individual needs. You should know that William works with the Spirit of Compassion to recommend the purest and most beneficial supplements available. I've since learned that the supplement market is big business, so make sure that you spend your money wisely.

5. *What are the healing benefits of celery juice?*

In addition to his Medical Medium book series, William is also the innovator of the global celery juice movement. In fact, his fifth book in his series is titled *Medical Medium Celery Juice: The Most Powerful Medicine of Our Time Healing Millions Worldwide*. He teaches that celery juice is the greatest healing tonic of all time, serving three main functions:

1. STRENGTHENS HYDROCHLORIC ACID (I.E., GOOD ACID) IN THE GUT

2. PROVIDES UNIQUE MINERAL SODIUM SALTS TO THE CENTRAL NERVOUS SYSTEM

3. AMBUSHES PATHOGENS

In addition, it's also helpful for acid reflux, for migraines, and for lowering your pathogen load, as well as being a more powerful tool for healing high cholesterol than a statin. The mineral sodium salt clusters, unique to celery juice, are known to break down the cell membranes of pathogens and rid the body of toxic acid from every crevice. I like to think of celery juice as a car detailing for the body.

Two days after I began reading *Medical Medium*, I bought a juicer and made my first glass of celery juice. On the fourth day of drinking it first thing in the morning, I noticed a strange smell in the car after dropping Sarah off at school. I then continued smelling it at home, while watching the Australian Open Tennis Tournament. The smell I recognized was just a faint aromatic memory from my childhood, until I suddenly realized that it smelled like ammonia. I smelled like Pine-Sol!

Apparently, I had low levels of hydrochloric acid in my gut due to viral infections, stress, and a congested liver. When this happens, dense protein-based foods like animal meat, nuts, and legumes can't be thoroughly digested. Instead, they rot and become rancid, creating ammonia gas in the gut. William has termed this condition "ammonia permeability." I had no idea this problem was inside of me.

The celery juice was transporting the ammonia out via my skin. Amazingly, I could literally smell progress! For over a month, I reeked of ammonia after drinking my celery juice. I even smelled like it during and after bathing. The celery juice was indeed moving the toxic gas out of my body.

One night, I felt an impending migraine. I drank a second celery juice, and within an hour, I was out of bed and functioning. I cooked dinner, cleaned the kitchen, and didn't retreat to my bedroom after dinner as usual. Instead, we watched *The Voice* in the living room and folded the laundry. Now celery juice didn't always make my migraines disappear so quickly, but I loved it when it did. (For more information about migraines, check out the chapter about migraines in the revised edition of *Medical Medium*.)

6. *Why are heavy metals such a health threat and where do they come from?*

William writes that toxic heavy metals (i.e., mercury, aluminum, copper, lead, nickel, arsenic, and cadmium) enter our bodies from numerous sources and gradually build up over time. We remain unaware, however, because we aren't taught about them, even though we often receive minor exposure to them.

Heavy metals are found in items we use in the kitchen, like cookware, drinkware, cutlery, aluminum foil, aluminum cans, tap water, seafood, foods with pesticides, foods cooked on an outdoor grill, pharmaceuticals, and recreational drugs. They are also found in bathroom items we use, like makeup, cosmetics, fluoride-containing toothpaste, hairspray, hair products, sunscreens, nail chemicals, talcum, and deodorants. You can also find these metals in the air as we breathe in chemtrails, fire-works, scented candles, chemical air fresheners, perfumes, and colognes. Other outside sources of heavy metals can be found in tattoo ink, dental work, tanning beds, dry-cleaning chemicals, cosmetic anti-wrinkle injections, other invasive cosmetic procedures, and nanotechnology sprays.

These toxic metals surround us, yet there is no proper way to measure our exposure to them. Current urine and blood tests are inaccurate because there's no proper way to measure the metals that seep into our organs, including our brains. Why is toxic metal removal from our bodies so important for our health? Because these heavy metals have been linked to the most significant physical and mental conditions we face today.

For example, *Medical Medium* boldly states, "No one likes Alzheimer's; it's a frightening, terrible disease. Yet it's rapidly becoming common—and it's 100 percent mercury-caused." William then adds that aluminum is commonly present in the brains of Alzheimer's patients along with mercury. Everyone on Earth has some undesirable metals hidden in their bodies.

When her extremely agitated white-haired mother was diagnosed with dementia, my friend asked me what she could do to avoid a dementia diagnosis herself. She researched William's Heavy Metal Detox Smoothie (HMDS) and began drinking it every morning. She's reported back that her brain fog has lifted, and she misses drinking the HMDS when she travels away from home.

Not only do we receive external exposure to toxic heavy metals, but William also explains that generations of toxic heavy metal accumulations are passed down through the bloodline. He blames mercury as an instigator of ADHD, autism, and most seizure disorders. Specifically, William adds that autism is a heightened form of ADHD caused by mercury and aluminum in the brain's cerebral midline canal (between the right and left hemispheres of the brain) and also in other parts of the brain. He encourages that these toxic heavy metals can be removed from a child's brain by using the tools and cleansing techniques written in Medical Medium. Early intervention may be best, as William explains that by early adulthood, the open space of the cerebral midline canal will close and trap the toxic heavy metals. His tools and cleansing techniques are available for any age to lessen the strain that interferes with life and relationships.

William states, "There's almost nothing better you can do for your health than to get heavy metals out of your body." He recommends drinking his HMDS daily to safely remove heavy metals from your body over time. You can find his recipe for this smoothie in his books and online. In time, I no longer needed my sauna treatments after adding the HMDS to my morning break-fast routine. (Hint: Cilantro is part of the HMDS. If you don't like the cilantro herb, use small amounts or omit it in the beginning.)

7. *What are the benefits of limiting or omitting fats from your diet?*

I first worked with two clients of William's who explained that it was important to cut out or limit animal protein and other fats (e.g., oils, nuts, legumes, and avocados), because fats clog the blood, the blood vessels, and the liver. This blockage makes it difficult for the liver to filter out all it must screen. They both told me that cleaner blood flow increases oxygen in the blood and allows more space in the blood vessels for the herbal supplements to travel throughout the body and get to work. William explains the constant intake of fatty foods induces an adrenaline rush to assist the liver in cleaning up the fat. Since our adrenal glands are overly stressed in today's society, lowering our fatty intake will give our organs a break. "Liquid gold" is how William defines adrenaline, and he encourages us to keep our adrenaline rushes to a minimum and preserve the helpful hormone for emergencies and safety. I *finally* understood why I needed to cut out the fats in my diet.

To understand how to heal chronic illness using the Medical Medium protocols, you must be willing to unlearn old agendas and learn to live a new way. In general, people freak out when you don't eat meat. They get extremely worried about you ingesting enough protein. William has an entire free SoundCloud podcast about it titled "Truth about Protein." Since the 1930s, the food industry has pushed the high protein diet, according to William, for the same reason any industry advertises a product—for mere profit. He further adds that the liver is responsible for creating the types of protein recognized by your body. He states the liver requires fruits, leafy greens, and vegetables to produce protein. It doesn't require eating the foods people think of as high in protein to produce protein. He adds that the trouble with the foods we associate with being high in protein (i.e., eggs, bacon, yogurt, beef, chicken, tofu, fish, milk, nuts, and seeds) is that they are also high in fat. He writes the truth is that proteins are found in all fruits and vegetables, so the protein options are endless. This was definitely new information to me!

Unfortunately, a high-protein/high-fat diet proved unhelpful in my case. Been there, done that, as they say. In fact, my high-fat diet, in addition to my lack of hydrochloric acid in my gut, was how I ended up smelling like Pine-Sol. William addresses the need to lower fat consumption precisely in *Liver Rescue*, the fourth book of his Medical Medium series. In it, he explains that a diet high in fat can lead to a toxic and sluggish liver, potentially resulting in heart attacks, strokes, and diabetes. When you eat a typical American diet filled with fats for every meal, it leaves the liver little time to do its two thousand critical chemical functions, according to William's *Liver Rescue* book.

This reminds me of the story I previously mentioned about a chiropractor who spoke about having a dinner party one night and never catching up on cleaning all the dishes. The benefit of omitting or limiting your fat intake is to allow your liver time to turn on its self-cleaning function. It's then that stored toxins of all types can be released, restoring your health and preventing future health issues. The environment can also benefit from a drop in beef intake, which would reduce methane and carbon dioxide gas emissions, conserve water, and slow down deforestation for cattle to roam and to grow their feed. Hint: For inspiration, check out the documentary *Live to 100: Secrets of the Blue Zones*, which highlights the places on Earth where people live the longest due to their low-fat diets.

8. Is true healing an individual sport?

I tried several times to increase my body's cleaning process, using some of the cleanses recommended in the Medical

Medium series, but I couldn't tolerate the deeper removal. It caused too much pain for me and my sensitivities. Some people can jump right into the cleanses and heal quickly, while others need to modify cleanses and realize that healing will be a process. The classic children's story "The Tortoise and the Hare" provides a moral lesson here, vividly showing us that "slow and steady wins the race." I was told if there is neurological involvement with your symptoms, you might be placed more in the category of a longer healing journey. That was definitely me. I bought a cute little blue and white wooden square sign reading, "Good Things Take Time," as a reminder to me to be patient. Patience is a trait needing practice, however.

During a phone appointment with one of the ladies I worked with, I complained, "I've already spent *five* years of grueling trials and errors trying to heal. How long is it going to take before I'm healthy again, before I get my life back?" That was the nagging question constantly on my mind.

"There is no magic time frame. Don't count the past five years. Realize you are working in a different way now and start paying attention to any changes because they may be subtle," she coached.

Boo, hiss, boo again! I preferred the magic. The time it takes to heal is an important factor to comprehend, though. I've heard the Medical Medium's methods have been criticized because the recommendations are universal, yet we are all different. However, we are both—different and the same. We have the same bodies with the same organs and systems functioning in the same way. It's why healing occurs for everyone.

Yet we are different in the types and amounts of addictions, toxins, and traumas we carry, and we need to be detoxed individually, at our own paces. The timing is different for everyone. It may seem that disease just appears one day following a scan, a blood test, or a lump. However, in reality, toxins become trapped in our bodies over time and eventually reveal themselves in various forms. Disease is grown over time and takes time to be disbanded.

9. *Why do more women than men suffer from chronic illness?*

Have you ever wondered why? What's the big difference between women and men having chronic illness? It boils down to our immune systems and a woman's reproductive cycle. In the Medical Medium series, the toll taken on a female's immune system during her reproductive cycle is revealed. It says that eighty percent of her immune system supports the reproductive system during menstruation, leaving only twenty percent to stand guard over the rest of her body. During ovulation, forty percent of her immune system supports the reproductive system, leaving only sixty percent to safeguard the rest of her body. While pregnant, fifty percent of the immune system supports the reproductive system and baby, leaving the other fifty percent to defend the rest of her body. During childbirth, over ninety percent of the immune system supports the reproductive system, leaving only ten percent to protect the rest of a woman's body.

In general, a woman's immune system needs more ammunition to stay healthy. This awareness highly encouraged me to dive into the Holy Five foods to help me heal and stave off any future illnesses. Hopefully, it encourages young women to do the same to prevent disease, adrenal fatigue, and post-partum depression.

10. *What's in your medication?*

It's widely accepted there are numerous side effects related to medications, but many people are dependent on their daily medications. In book seven of the Medical Medium series, *Brain Saver*, I was shocked to learn that big industries have secretly merged into our medication supply. William and the SOC revealed that since the 1940s and 1950s, caffeine has been added to nearly all pharmaceuticals as an ingredient. That addition certainly isn't helping the caffeine addiction so prevalent today. He states caffeine harms us in two distinct ways—it dehydrates us and stresses the adrenal glands to release adrenaline as if you are in a crisis situation. He adds that caffeine addiction can lead to premature aging, damaged skin, brain fog, concentration problems, fatigue, hair loss, and weight gain.

Besides caffeine, I was startled to hear that all pharmaceuticals also contain some level of toxic heavy metals. How ironic, because the toxic heavy metals are partially responsible for disease to begin with! William writes, "we may find ourselves on medications for extended periods of time, with the medications possibly making our conditions worse."

As all the new information I had learned settled in, I quit my bee venom therapy after learning the stings triggered the Lyme disease viruses. First thing every morning, I drank lemon water with honey. Then fifteen to thirty minutes later, I juiced and drank fresh celery juice. Another fifteen to thirty minutes later, I drank the HMDS. My morning remained fat-free, giving my liver the chance to continue its nightly self-cleaning duties. (You can find a version of this morning routine in the fifth book of the Medical Medium series, *Cleanse to Heal,* and on social media.)

Following my morning routine, I ate a salad for lunch with homemade dressing (without oil or vinegar) or a drizzle of honey and included a few adrenal fatigue snacks every one to two hours. Adrenal fatigue snacks are a combination of glucose (fruit), sodium (leafy green), and potassium (piece of banana, date, honey, or other food high in potassium). An example could be a piece of apple, a celery stick, and a date. (You can find more examples on William's website.) By eating these mini snacks every few hours, you can prevent the blood sugar dips we often feel every afternoon. That's the time when I used to reach for a piece of chocolate or an unproductive sugar or caffeine source to keep me going. Now, I no longer have those afternoon slumps.

Each day I drank various medicinal herbal teas, ate cooked veggies and potatoes with a salad for dinner and fruit for dessert, if I desired. I ate raw and fat-free/low-fat foods until 4:00 P.M. or all day, and I took supplements as recommended. There was no eating out, and so much of my day consisted of grocery shopping, food prep, and cooking. The other parts of my day, besides my typical chores, were filled with detoxing via yoga (if possible), walking, rebounding, massage, reflexology, sleeping, and using my infrared sauna. Healing is a job!

Six months into this new way of healing, I was riddled with another onslaught of issues. Some were the same, while others were new ones like frozen shoulder, tinnitus, dry eyes, eye floaters, quarter-sized red itchy welts, and massive migraines. To this day, I still cannot tolerate chemical fragrances and had to stop going to reflexology appointments because their office began using plug-in scents. William teaches chemical fragrances are worse than cigarettes for our lungs.

William's client also told me I had a high viral load, high neurologic stress load, high heavy metal load, and a sluggish lymph system. She also mentioned it was normal to feel uncomfortable as I detoxed. Then she instructed me to slowly increase the intake of some of my supplements for a boost. Within three days of increasing them, I was extremely irritated, both physically and mentally. My supplement ingestion increase had elevated my neurotoxic pain. I crashed, taking a long nap and waking to feeling broken as if I was in a hundred pieces. When I found myself yelling at Fluffy for tangling her leash around my legs on the walking path, I *knew* something had to give. So, I reduced my supplement intake to a manageable dosage. It was a callback to taking an active role and advocating for myself.

To make matters worse, my own family members ridiculed my diet. My mom would try a dish I made for myself then say, "That tastes like cardboard." My dad made nasty-nose-

 Making a Way

squinched-and-tongue-out "yuck" faces at my celery juice. Frannie would "rescue" Sarah from having to eat dinner with us and take her out to eat, as they both made their own "yuck" faces toward the kitchen. Often, Sarah would fill up on junk food prior to dinner, although I was cooking two separate meals at that time. John continued thinking everything was okay in moderation and was continually frustrated with my inconvenient food issues, while not budging with his food choices. If I said something to the kids like, "You should eat an apple a day," Evan used deflection. He'd respond with, "Okay, I'll have three milkshakes a day, Mama."

When Patrick was younger, he insisted straightforwardly on "proof" of any dietary choices I encouraged. But I didn't have valid answers for him then because I hadn't read *Medical Medium,* and I wasn't a vision of health yet. He became known as Organic Patrick via his friends after they raided our pantry and saw what he brought to school in his lunch box.

Our kids just wanted to eat what their friends were eating and what was attractive to their taste buds—the typical American diet. But as I was learning about all the harmful troublemaker foods, I also desperately wanted to protect them. I didn't want them to ever have the issues I was having. I wanted to undo the dietary habits we had instilled and teach new ones. I had every reason to let go of the old eating habits, but they did not. They always proclaimed, "We don't have any food in this house!" and "We are already healthy!" Sarah even grew up thinking "organic" was a bad thing. I wished I had used Ahmed's lesson for her children: One night, she put a bottle of pesticide on the dinner table and asked who would like some on their food. Her three girls hurriedly refused!

A wall of separation continued to exist between me and the rest of my family. I was in one space, and they were in another. I spent more time alone and in prayer. A regular counselor wouldn't have understood this ongoing twilight zone, so counseling wasn't an option. I had little energy to give relationships. My energy was reserved for my healing and my kids, as a means of protecting them and trying to be a normal mom. I realized I had to lean on my faith harder, stronger, tighter.

I remained stuck between two worlds: the normal world and the barriers of a chronic illness. I understood God was urging me to make more time for the latter of the two. Singer Lauren Daigle sang out and reminded me to "Look Up Child." I favored her familiar Cajun accent and jazzy roots. I drew on forgiveness for the family's teasing, yet I loved my family anyway, even when I felt their resistance. My love was innate. Sometimes in life we have to make choices for ourselves that may not be popular with those we love. I focused on God having prosperous plans for me and never letting me go. As I tried to fall asleep each night, I pictured Mother Mary embracing me in her loving arms as we rocked in the palm of His hand.

"For I know the plans I have for you, plans to prosper you and give you a future," Jeremiah 29:11.

CHAPTER 10

Fork in the Road

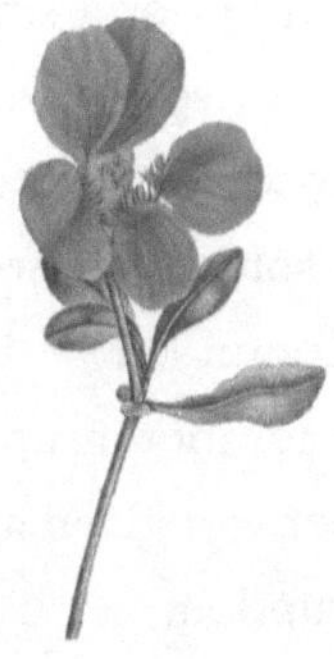

FOR SEVERAL WEEKS, I was ambushed by the onslaught of symptoms during the night. I abandoned my marital bed and moved to Patrick's empty bed without waking John. I was losing hope of this condition ever dissipating. I had days when all I thought about was standing in front of a bus or a nearby train. Just when I was at the end of my personal resources for my own support, I joined online classes led by Muneeza Ahmed (one of Anthony William's sought-after clients who shares his Medical Medium information).

Her classes were titled "Intuitive Cleanse" and "Detox Mastery." The cleanse was a two-week class, while the mastery class was three months long. She created the mastery class as a program to help save others, as she was saving herself. Both classes included a variety of printable handouts, but my favorites were the clean salad dressing recipes free of oil and vinegar. The classes offered teaching webinars, Q&A webinars, a wellness journal, recipes, emails, case studies, and tons of support. I barely knew how to use Facebook, and my computer skills were low, not to mention the brain fog I was experiencing, but I muddled through as best I could.

Muneeza had us sign up for a small group. Members were located all over the world, so you had to choose a time zone that worked for your schedule. I was amazed at how many people, mostly women but some men, were taking the classes. My small group met via Zoom, before it became so popular. We "gathered" once a week for moral support in a safe space free of judgment. Each member was given an allotted amount of time to speak without interruption.

In our group, Nelly introduced herself: "I'm in the northeast, and it is snowing today. I've been following AW [William] for about a year. I'm an artist at heart but also a health coach. I feel so much better when I stay off the no-foods, but occasionally I eat them without too much discomfort. I'm trying to teach my husband to eat better too, but he prefers my old way of cooking, and my family doesn't take any health-related suggestions I offer. They prefer to go to a doctor."

Another member, Stacy, opened by saying, "I've been following Anthony for a couple of years. I was taking a class in functional medicine, but I stopped because there were so many contradictions with what Anthony teaches. I've battled Lyme disease fatigue, depression, and infertility. I stick to the no-foods for the most part. I've taken all of Muneeza's programs, and I really enjoy her. I'm trying to help my son get better with the protocols because he can hardly eat."

Anne, another member, vocalized, "I'm in New Mexico, and it's hot here! I've had symptoms my whole life in retrospect, after reading *Medical Medium*. I was a sickly kid, and now my kids struggle. I see how the viruses and heavy metals are passed down from generation to generation. I've had fertility issues and pregnancy issues. I used IVF for my children. When they were young, I couldn't function, couldn't walk, and had multiple anaphylactic reactions. I was diagnosed with muscular dystrophy and needed a walker. I read the book and changed my entire diet to comply with the Medical Medium information. There was a huge difference in the first few weeks and months that followed. I no longer needed the walker, and my balance was much better. My children and siblings each have issues that Medical Medium addresses, so I'm working with them to get healthier. Hopefully, they will comply. I'm so grateful for this information!"

Soft-spoken member Cindy shared, "I've had health problems for many years. They started when I was a kid. I had visits to the ER, but the doctors always said nothing was wrong with me. Now, I have hypothyroidism and adrenal fatigue. I've been searching for answers for a long time, and I started using Medical Medium info eight months ago. My husband says he has seen a difference, but he doesn't want to make changes in his diet. I have to cook for him separately. We live remotely, so I spend time driving a good distance to get organic foods. And it is so time-consuming to do the Medical Medium protocols. No one believes my symptoms."

I shared my story with them. I was thrilled to meet these women. We were all at the start of something new, and we had so much in common. None of our husbands had an interest in this transformative information. I learned the value of actively listening and the need to be supported for healing. I had finally found my tribe! I began to *believe* I could heal.

Muneeza insisted passionately and repeatedly, "ALL CHRONIC ILLNESS CAN HEAL!" She *saw* us! She was also a client of William's for many years and was sharing what she learned as a client about applying the Medical Medium information. She was breaking down the Medical Medium tools and answers to empower us to do our own healing. The lesson and permission to use self-love and self-compassion opened my heart even wider. This beautiful woman met with individual clients as well, and one day she shared that her sixteen-year-old client wished she were hospitalized, so people would believe she was sick. We understood. The mystery illnesses are rampant and affecting every age group.

Muneeza's passion was contagious and amplified my belief and ability to heal myself. I'm mostly grateful for two things. Anne and Cindy still speak with me via Zoom. They both teach me so much and act as a sounding board for life and for all things Medical Medium–related. And I am grateful for the lesson to release being the *victim* in order to become the *victor*. I didn't realize I had felt like a victim until Muneeza spoke the word. The sudden realization helped me release the notion and make space for becoming victorious.

I experienced a shift. I had more energy, less fatigue, less pain, a newfound hope, and no more suicidal thoughts. I *finally* had answers that made sense and had real support and compassion. I no longer felt alone. There continued to be days and weeks when I felt better. There also continued to be many things I couldn't attend. Besides normal daily outings, I missed weddings and family reunions. There also continued to be pain and prayer in my life. But me being the victim was gone, and the *victor was rising.*

Although the process took me one step forward and then two steps back, I still had amazing news to report. In a six-year period, I had likely driven an hour away and back less than five times. The stars finally aligned, however, and I was able to drive myself three and a half hours from home to Evan's competition. With it being his senior year, I didn't want to miss out on supporting his endeavor. I knew my time was limited with him before he began college.

Traveling was a stretch for me, yet doors opened. As her last deeply valued service to our family, Amber came over to cook so I had dinner meals ready to go. I eagerly shopped for my breakfast routine and arranged salads for lunch. I cut salad fixings into small glass jars so they could easily be topped onto a bed of lettuce, then crowned with a clean homemade dressing—great for on the go! Evan's competitions were scheduled during the afternoons, so I had plenty of time for my morning concoctions.

John didn't have to travel for work, so he would be home with Sarah, and my friend was able to bring her home from school. Off I went with my car filled with everything but my kitchen sink. I had a juicer, a Vitamix, an electric tea kettle, jugs of spring water, a bag of supplements, and a set of sheets to replace scented hotel sheets. My ice chest was filled with food, wooden utensils, a cutting board, a ceramic knife, paper products, dish soap, and a sponge. I learned the Vitamix and the juicer had to be washed in the bathtub since they wouldn't fit in the little sink. I adapted to a hotel room, and my food fit perfectly in the small hotel refrigerator we had arranged with the front desk to have in the room.

It was quite the operation, but well worth it, because this adventure was the largest miracle yet on my healing journey. I was even able to walk on a treadmill without getting dizzy. I found a penny as I walked to the competition across the street. I knew my angels were nearby. Evan and his team were nervous, so I texted him Bob Marley's song "Three Little Birds," messaging him not to worry. On days like this, it was easier to step into timelessness instead of needing to know how long it would take to be completely healed. I was grateful to celebrate this triumph and freedom with John over the phone, and I was learning to be patient with my setbacks.

There was a time when I thought my alternate-eating-for-health pattern was only going to be a part-time gig. Yet, I had changed, and I'd learned to ride a new bike, so to speak. I found the best, most efficient, shiniest, most promising bike out there, complete with all the bells and whistles. I was learning a new Medical Medium language, which I couldn't unlearn because it was saving my life. I was also learning a new way to approach health issues, and I saw great potential for myself and others.

One evening following a soccer game, I witnessed a female student lying on the cement in the middle of the parking lot. I was extremely alarmed. I wondered if she'd passed out or needed an ambulance. The nurse in me contemplated possible physical health issues. Later, I spoke with the principal, who informed me the student was having a panic attack. He said it happened every day during the school day and was a common occurrence.

Anxiety and depression are rampant in an epidemic of their own. Last year alone, three friends who've taken anti-anxiety and anti-depressive medications for many years were diagnosed with cancer. I hear more and more young people nowadays are on those medications due to their crippling anxiety and depression. It is taking over their lives, leaving them powerless and unable to perform normal daily tasks. I remember a commercial in the nineties with Susan Powter calling out, "Stop the insanity." Her message was about losing weight naturally by eating low-fat and moving your body. But her message to "stop the insanity" still rings true today for gaining our health back in mind, body, and spirit as an entire society. William has a different take on anxiety and depression, as outlined in his *Medical Medium Brain Saver* duo book set. I kept seeing physical and mental health issues in every direction I turned. I saw the widespread potential to implement William's protocols to heal and prevent chronic illness.

I kept going. I was doing everything to reduce heavy metals in my body and toxins in our home. I changed all of my household-cleaning products. My personal products changed to fluoride-free toothpaste, aluminum-free deodorant, and, fortunately, I'd never used hairspray. I also stopped using candles and anything with fragrances, replacing them with beeswax candles from the local farmer's market and a diffuser for essential oils. Over time, we acquired organic mattresses and organic cotton sheets. I slowly acquired ceramic-coated pots, pans, knives, and peelers, in addition to wooden kitchen utensils and plates without lead or cadmium. I began using glass instead of plastic whenever possible and switched to using parchment paper instead of aluminum foil. I never drink out of aluminum cans and use aluminum-canned food goods very seldom. My seafood intake had ceased, and I was already buying organic foods with less pesticides than conventional foods. I felt I was divinely being pulled deeper and deeper into learning about the new methods and recipes, all without knowing what the future held for us.

One day out of the blue, John's dad gave me a call to check on me. This was unusual, as he wasn't a fan of using the phone at all—a man of few words. Frannie usually made all the phone calls. We had a nice conversation, and I assured him I was doing okay, even though I was having a hard time. It was easy to pretend over the phone that I was fine and not cause him to worry. John's mom called unexpectedly a few weeks later, saying his dad had just passed from a heart attack in their home, while he was rocking in his favorite chair. We were all in shock. John and his brother quickly packed and drove out of state. My boys drove Sarah and me to meet them as soon as possible. We stayed at a hotel near their home. The funeral services were long because Big John, as we called him, had worked in the banking industry at the same bank his entire life. In addition, he had lived in the same city his entire life. He had built numerous relationships over his lifetime, and many wanted to pay their respects.

After the services, we moved out of the hotel and into their home because the hotel was chock-full of scented fragrances that affected me terribly. I was supposed to be supporting my husband, mother-in-law, and family, yet the emotional and physical difficulty took its toll on me. By the evening, I had a terrible migraine and couldn't get out of bed, so I skipped dinner and lay as still as possible. John brought me water, supplements, an Advil, and a cold washcloth to lay over my forehead. The next morning, Frannie saw me walking gingerly and wearing sunglasses and said she thought they were going to have to call an ambulance for me the night before.

I don't like to be the problem. I was a nurse; I want to be part of the solution—the helper. Frannie was cooking breakfast for everyone instead of being allowed to get on with the grieving process, which made me feel even worse. Our hearts were broken. I still treasure my last phone conversation with Big John and am grateful for all the church candles he lit on my behalf as a prayer for healing.

Unfortunately, there were more ways that I wasn't keeping up with my wifely and motherly duties. So, John and I opted for a weekend away. The location was based on a Whole Foods grocery store and a health market/juice bar being nearby. I was assured I'd have access to organic produce. However, the trip turned quickly sour. I had a migraine lasting several days, and it was rainy. I only went outside for two hours during the three days we were there, and I cried at church, pleading to God for mercy to reduce the pain. John's vacation was ruined! We deduced that the building must have been moldy, triggering my Lyme disease viruses into a flare.

We had made it home when I had another migraine that lasted four days after taking a chance on salmon from a local eatery. I knew better than to eat mercury-laden seafood, but I craved something new for my palate and didn't want to cook. Once again, I had to lie still because I was too dizzy to walk around. The only good thing about the migraine was escaping into a book by Elin Hilderbrand and reading about someone else's drama. The advice from *Medical Medium* had resonated with me, and I could read for pleasure once again.

John and I spontaneously decided to try another beach trip to reconnect as a family before the boys were both away at college. There is nothing a mom wants deeper than peace, love, and joy among her family. I used to be the glue that kept us together. We were away for a brief five days, half of which I stayed inside the condo. I remember forcing myself to go to the beach and being very dizzy. I felt the burden of how my maladies disconnected the family unit, and I felt their frustration. I thought educating them would aid in their understanding. I encouraged them to eat better foods to promote their immune systems. Yet, no one was interested, and I still sounded like a broken record. They followed John's lead, which was to ignore any nutrition advice I suggested and eat whatever they wanted. *She's crazy*, they must've thought. By the time I got to the Medical Medium advice, John and the kids had mentally checked out.

I ran into a friend at the grocery store. "Hi, how are you doing?" I asked.

"We are doing fine! We just got back from Las Vegas, and all the boys are working until school starts," she answered. "How are the Kellys?"

"It's been a rough summer! We lost John's dad in June. It was sudden. The kids are all keeping busy and getting ready for another semester. I've been struggling physically. Sometimes, I wonder if John will leave me," I confided.

"Well, you are lucky he hasn't left you!" she retorted nonchalantly.

Did she really say that? It hit me like a bag of bricks, mentally and emotionally knocking me down! The following day was our twenty-third wedding anniversary, yet it didn't feel celebratory. When you feel like you have the flu all the time, you have zero libido. I remembered a few things from our church's premarital classes. In those classes, an experienced couple taught the young couples how women were like irons when it came to being romantic, needing time to warm up. But that men were like light switches, able to turn it on and off at the drop of a hat. They encouraged the young couples to be best friends and to hear one another. They taught that women felt heard through long conversations and men felt heard through sex. It's interesting how some lessons stick with you over many years. Neither of us was feeling heard.

At one point I said to John, "I'm healing myself from two incurable diseases."

He laughed and said, "Yeah, right."

What did he think I was doing? "You aren't willing to change anything, are you?" I frustratingly asked.

"What *have* you changed?" he asked, attempting to turn it around.

"What *haven't* I changed? I've changed everything down to my toothpaste!" I exclaimed.

He had no further arguing remarks.

I began envisioning what it would look like if we parted ways. Sara Bareilles's song "Brave" taught me to be brave and say what I needed to say. It became clear to me that the most difficult discussions are with the ones you care the most about. One cold and quiet morning, John and I were sitting by the fireplace, drinking our morning drinks. He was nursing a cup of black coffee, and I was sipping a glass mug of lemon water with a teaspoon of honey.

"I feel like our love is gone. I feel like we don't love each other anymore," I sadly disclosed.

He sat there, taken aback. "What are you talking about? What do you mean?"

"I know you pretend to support the Medical Medium adaptations, but you are so skeptical. I asked you to read the book about Lyme and the *Medical Medium* book. You say you'll read them, but you haven't," I said.

"I've read some things," he replied.

"I've been looking at other places to live, although it already feels like we are separated in our marriage, in our own home. We seem to be ignoring each other. I don't think you want any part of this new lifestyle I'm living, and that's okay. I'm not holding you hostage. I know I hold you back, and I don't want to do that anymore. You deserve to live the life you want, not the life you feel obligated to live. You can go live a normal life, and I'll surround myself with sincere support."

"But I think we need to work on this," he decided.

So, we took baby steps. We started reading a devotional book filled with short stories of couples who had been married for over fifty years. We were hoping to gain wisdom via osmosis from their experiences, but we soon realized that we had to work it out on our own. John dreamed of doing normal couple activities, while I dreamed of being symptom-free. He suggested couples therapy. Did I want another health professional judging me and my symptoms? Absolutely not! But I agreed to try it. We had one joint session with the therapist, which was mostly informational about our circumstances. It was the most uneasy emotional situation I've ever had. Then we went to separate sessions with her.

I went first. "I know I'm leading a different lifestyle, but I've accepted it for my survival," I honestly expressed. "My family doesn't like it, and they don't participate. They don't understand what I'm doing. Now, we aren't eating the same meals at all. Every day they eat this, and I eat that. The next day, they eat this, and I eat that, and so on. It creates an even greater separation, and I think John blames me for all of it," I told her.

"So, you are okay with yourself and your life right now? And, you know you can't change anyone but yourself?" she asked.

"Yes," I spoke.

"I don't think we need another session then."

"Oh, thank goodness!"

It was John's turn. He had two private sessions with her. He said, "She was very helpful. She did a good job of helping me realize things I said and did weren't supporting you. She taught me I was stuck on the life we *had*, but all couples change over time, with or without chronic illness. Then she mentioned I had to decide what I wanted."

We both had much to process and choices to make. We had a lot at stake. The therapy was more beneficial than I'd expected. The therapist brought our issues to the surface. We were at a fork in the road. Time and space were our allies.

I held onto William's statement about the chronically ill: "You are not to blame for your illness. It's not something you manifested or attracted. It's not your fault. You certainly don't deserve to feel unwell. You have a God-given right to heal." His words soaked into my thirsty soul. I didn't know why our lives had been disrupted. I just knew I had to keep going and that maybe I needed my own space, free of blame, to truly heal.

On the way home from an outing, our family of five stopped for lunch. The teenagers teased me for bringing my lunch into the restaurant. I was triggered and defensive, so I told the boys to date girls who eat healthy. Patrick had started speaking to a girl named Amy. Honestly, I worried about the future and adding more people to our family who wouldn't comprehend my eating style. *Would the divide grow?* I worried about being the grandparent who doesn't give my grandkids processed foods and candy but invites them into the kitchen to make healthier treats. They might still prefer the bad stuff, and I'll love them too much for it. I learned to hold a place of wellness for my loved ones, because who knows when and if they'll ever decide to eat more fruits and vegetables and learn what they are putting into their bodies. I learned to respect their choices, and in return, have them respect mine. Respect is key to harmony.

The kids wanted to eat the typical American diet, just like their friends. Sarah wanted lots of refined sugar, pizza, ice cream, gum, and chemical-laden cosmetics. Patrick and Evan were into frozen dinners and fast food while in college. My cooked meals couldn't compete with all the addictive fillers, fats, monosodium glutamate (MSG), and sodium they were consuming in restaurants and processed foods. I had eaten the same way in college because I had no idea how harmful those foods could be or how many illnesses they'd feed.

During one visit from my parents, they commented they couldn't do what I was doing and eat like I was eating. I replied if they hurt like I did, they could do it. I was concerned about their health, as my mom battled breast cancer and diverticulitis. My dad's health issues had intensified, with a trip to the ER for a severe bout of vertigo and nausea. He was alarmed when a scan showed he'd had a stroke at some point in the past. The hospital staff then regulated his blood pressure medications and explained that his positive antinuclear antibody (ANA) blood test revealed inflammation and possibly lupus. Nothing definitive was decided from the ANA test results, although he continued having joint pain along with other symptoms.

My parents watched how John and Sarah began drinking fruit smoothies for breakfast. John had started drinking smoothies after watching *The Game Changers* documentary with me. It highlights professional athletes at the top of their game who eat primarily plant-based diets. We had never seen anything like it.

Like most Americans, we were reared on meat as the main course with other foods on the side. It's a different mindset to eat fruits and vegetables as both the main course and the sides. My parents decided they might start having fruit smoothies for breakfast, on occasion, as well. Everyone gets to decide, everyone has choices, and all the choices are correct for each person on their own journey. I was reminded by my friends Anne and Cindy how important it is to allow everyone to make their own choices in life because that is how each soul grows.

One of my aunts told me a story following my uncle's death, as she recalled their years together. She said every time she would visit her sister an hour away, my uncle would yell at her to leave early. On a recent trip to visit her sister, she began her journey home later than usual and got caught in traffic, arriving home in the dark. She realized that my uncle had never told her he was worried about her on the road. He didn't explicitly show her his care. Instead, he yelled demandingly, triggering her defenses. With reflection, she comprehended he was taking care of her the only way he knew how. Since then, she's rediscovered many other ways he showed her love, normal things a spouse handles that we may take for granted. Without knowing, my aunt had helped me rediscover many ways that John cared for me and the kids. She helped me realize couples with different perspectives could co-exist. *Maybe our soul connection could be restored, and we could build a new life together?*

We had watched the *Heal* documentary. "What did you think?" I asked him when it was over.

"They are saying there is power in *believing* you can heal," he answered.

"Along the way, you stopped believing I could heal, and I feel your doubt," I said.

Yet shortly after watching it, his attitude changed and his faith in healing seemed renewed. While John spent more time envisioning his future, I continued building a better me. Things were better between us, yet still fragile.

I read God answered prayers in three ways: Yes, No, and Not Yet. It was difficult to know if I was making progress. I felt I was still in the Not Yet category. There were highs and lows on this journey. At the beginning of 2019, I celebrated two years straight of drinking celery juice every morning. I was healing from the inside out, but my outside wasn't an exhibit of health. In a two-year period, I had gained over thirty pounds while eating cleaner than anyone I knew. I was only eating raw fruits and vegetables until 4:00 P.M. and then ate cooked veggies for dinner. I avoided all the foods on the Medical Medium's no-foods list, along with fats from meat, oils, and nuts. *What was happening?* I was eating fruits and vegetables and gaining weight.

The weight gain on this healing plan went against everything I had learned about weight issues. I thought one's weight reflected what they ate and their activity level. In the *Medical Medium Liver Rescue*, the fourth book in the series, William explains in Chapter 12 that "most of the time—an overwhelming amount of time—weight gain is really about the liver. While two other factors, the thyroid and the adrenals, can often be involved, it's important to remember that they both lead back to the liver." He writes that a viral load, adrenal strain, and toxic exposure are factors burdening the liver and decreasing the liver's ability to act as your filter.

Furthermore, he states, "weight is about the troublemaker storage department of the liver—for a person who can eat what she wants and not gain weight, it hasn't been compromised yet." We, as a society, assume if someone is slim and trim, they are healthy. However, we cannot see the exact function of their brain, heart, circulation, or any other organ or system in their body. Are we assuming incorrectly? By incorporating the Medical Medium information, could one take their weight issues into their own hands while cleaning their livers, instead of giving attention to the weight loss industry and possibly adding to their toxic load? William warns in his "Ditch the Weight Loss Drugs for Peaches & Nectarines & How to Make a Peach Pie Milkshake" YouTube episode that in five to ten years, the damages of the current weight loss drugs will begin to show themselves. He adds that no one needs these drugs when they learn that healthy weight loss happens from repairing the organs in our bodies.

Years before finding the Medical Medium healing truths, I learned that my liver was in jeopardy, and now I'd finally found the tools to set it free and regain my health. Fortunately, Muneeza explained in a teaching Zoom call exactly why my weight gain was happening. Without fats to filter, my liver was able to enlarge its self-cleaning capacity. As it was cleaning out my toxic load, it needed a place to store the toxins until I could safely excrete them. My body intuitively held on to enough fat content to act as a protective storage facility of sorts. It was amazing to experience a phenomenon that I never knew existed in my own body. The weight was undeniably uncomfortable, yet this journey had never been about weight; it had been about retrieving my health. Muneeza taught me to "Love your fat because it is saving your life!" Bet you've never heard that one before!

I tried to make the best of it. I have always been pear-shaped, but suddenly I was pear- *and* apple-shaped. I was a *papple*! My stomach had always been flat and my hips wide, so it was strange to witness the added fat around my middle and back, right near my liver. When I outgrew my comfy, stretchy, next-size-up clothes, it was time to make a trip to the maternity store. Sarah came with me to the mall. She went next door to shop for a bikini, while I explained to the maternity store workers that I had a medical condition causing my stomach to protrude. It was very disheartening!

To my surprise, the salesperson didn't bat an eye, replying, "So many ladies come to the store for all kinds of reasons. All of the girls who work here wear the clothes because they are so much more comfortable."

Her words immediately set me at ease yet reinforced the sadness I have for the masses struggling with weight. I'd been an overweight child who went to a diet center for assistance in second grade. She led me around the store, gathering basics for me to try on in the dressing room. Two things came to mind: The dressing room mirrors displayed a very humble picture, and the young lady was spot on. The clothes were definitely much more comfortable! I kept reminding myself that my weight gain was temporary. My day was filled with a high of finding comfy clothes to wear and a low of going home to prepare my salad dressing while my husband sat at the dining table eating his Italian takeout.

I did get tired of shopping for, cutting, and cooking food every single day and being careful with everything I ate. Prior to the mall excursion, I'd eaten a few bites of store-bought hummus, which left my nervous system buzzing overnight. If I ventured off my safe foods list at all, it resulted in me being in some sort of pain. I reached out to Muneeza to address it. I asked her about California poppyseed, a non-narcotic and non-addictive pain supplement listed at the Medical Medium Amazon store. She suggested I begin by taking four a day. Two weeks later, I increased the dose to six a day after waking up every two hours in pain for two straight nights. It was then that I slept through the night for the first time in years. I realized I should've been on this supplement a long time ago, as pain causes an adrenaline rush that feeds the viruses. Pain takes a toll on the body, inhibiting healing. Eight capsules a day of California poppyseed for me worked to keep the edge off.

John noticed I needed some help. He offered to make my applesauce, steam brussels sprouts, and chop salad vegetables, all without me asking. We were side by side in the kitchen as I prepared a potato dish. I know it isn't easy on family members of the chronically ill. Support goes a long way, and every tomorrow has room to enjoy a better day. My husband and I had turned in the same direction at the fork in the road. We'd both changed and met at the invisible line in the sand. Along the way, I gained valuable resources of friendship, counseling, understanding, confidence, and comfortable clothes. My eyes were opened to these phrases: "You can heal," "You are not to blame," "Self-love," "Self-compassion," and "Goodbye victim, hello victor."

CHAPTER 11

In Sickness and in Health

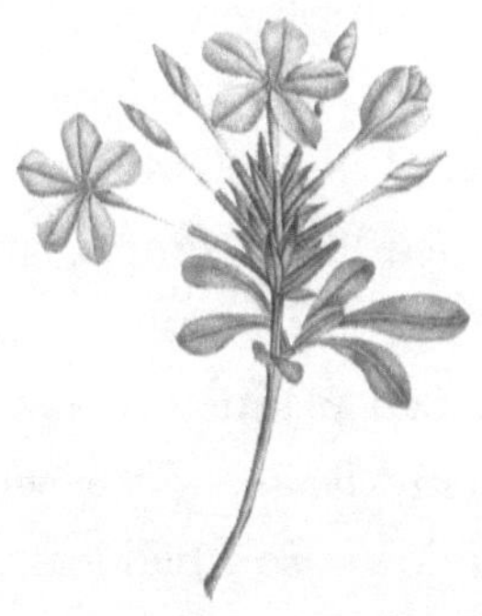

PROGRESS WAS SLOW AND often took a few steps backward. My new small group of friends connected me with a counselor familiar with the Medical Medium information. I was relaxed and unintimidated by her as we spoke on the phone. She addressed keeping my diet vibrant by eating the rainbow, answered questions I had about some supplements, and encouraged me to do extra juicing by adding in an afternoon celery or cucumber juice. She taught me to keep praying for my family to rise to new heights together so we could live in harmony. She introduced me to Donna Eden's daily energy exercises live on YouTube. These online exercises were easy, free, quick, and not another supplement I had to ingest. Of all the things I tried, this one stuck. I now have the exercises memorized and still frequently do them.

Lastly, this counselor explained that the solar flares from the sun coincided with the bedridden days I'd had. I had never heard of a solar flare before. NASA states a solar flare occurs when magnetic energy, which has built up in the solar atmosphere, is suddenly released. The amount of energy released is the equivalent of millions of one-hundred-megaton hydrogen bombs exploding at the same time! Apparently, this isn't something seen but felt. I learned I needed to give myself a lot of grace.

I pushed my limits, though, when John and I rented a boat on a nearby lake. We were striving to branch out a little bit, and boating seemed like a simple outing. I knew it was risky, and the following day I paid the price and was stuck in bed all day. John had planned to take me car shopping, but those plans quickly flew out the window. Disappointment was always a letdown, so I had learned not to make any plans. During weeks like those, I was reminded to dig deep as my own advocate and caretaker amid my family's needs, confusion, and skepticism. One evening, I was emptying the dishwasher in my robe. Evan and his jolly group of friends walked in the kitchen side door unexpectedly. They would always sit down on the kitchen barstools and visit with me as they came and went. But that night I had no words—nothing left to give. There simply wasn't enough energy to deal with everything and everyone, so I retreated to my bed until I was restored enough to continue onward. It was the best I could do then. I simply didn't have any more tears to cry. I had cried them all already. I was waiting on the Lord to respond and divine timing for healing. I tried to focus on gratitude, while often living in the reality of sadness and solitude. I remembered what it felt like to be normal, and I was working every day wholeheartedly to fully return home.

At the end of June 2019, my family arrived home from Breckenridge, Colorado. They'd been on a summer mountain vacation filled with adventures of mountain biking, white water rafting, fly-fishing, and zip-lining. The week before they left, I prayed for answers as to whether I should go with them or stay home. The answer was clear because my days leading up to the trip were filled with pain and fatigue. I was *so* angry! As I've said before, the worst part was missing out on spending time with my family. Boy, was I angry I'd be left behind, with them in Colorado and me back at home.

It took me a few days to work past it, as I spent time outside on the back patio glider and took short, soothing walks under the trees. From my devotional book, *Jesus Calling*, I absorbed, "Stay on the high road with Me. Many voices clamor for your attention, trying to divert you to another path. But I have called you to walk ever so closely with Me, soaking in My Presence, living in My Peace." The night before they left, I felt an immense sense of tranquility. Once the car was loaded with their suitcases, I led the five of us in prayer. I thanked God for a fun and refreshing time for them, and for the wisdom to know I needed more time to heal. Their stress was relieved, and their excitement was mounting. I was happy they could enjoy this opportunity. While they were away, all the energy I had was poured into taking care of myself, and I learned it was more time-consuming than I realized. I appreciated the time and space to retreat because I needed it.

The rest of the summer remained stagnant for me. John and the kids moved Frannie into an apartment while her new home was being built. I was unable to physically travel and help her move, but I sent a bag of move-in necessities, including paper towels, toilet paper, hand soap, bottled water, and so on. I was desperately hoping to see breakthroughs with my health. I wanted so badly for something to change. I became obsessed with following local realty listings. It allowed me to dream of external elation while sitting at my computer.

Physically, I had reached another low and felt like a balloon about ready to pop. I had no energy, and my feet hurt terribly, so poor Fluffy hadn't been for a walk in months. I was rocking a natural look without makeup, because I'd grown sensitive to even organic makeup, likely due to their heavy metals. Eye makeup and wearing contacts caused migraines, so I was always sporting my eyeglasses. I didn't see the ice on our white tiled floor, which had fallen from our extra refrigerator in the laundry room. I slipped on ice and fell to the ground awkwardly, breaking the last two toes on my right foot. The next day, Patrick bumped into me and stepped on those same two toes. When the toes began to heal, I'd repeatedly hit them accidentally. Finally, I purchased an orthopedic shoe to protect my right foot. Nothing was changing, and I had slowed down even further in my healing.

Meanwhile, life was moving right along for our kids. Patrick lived at home for the summer, working nine-to-five at an engineering internship for a power company. We were glad to have his positive spirit home before his senior year of college. He had a huge appetite but didn't cook, so there was more work for this tired mama. At twenty-two years old, he was full of energy and couldn't comprehend chronic fatigue. Pain and chronic fatigue are invisible yet take a toll on the masses. Patrick kept his social calendar rolling with friends and girlfriend visits from Amy, going to the gym, rock climbing, and attending bible studies.

He and Amy met through one of Patrick's roommates. Amy was a wiz in the kitchen and may have wooed Patrick over her macaroni and cheese. Their faith drew them into a deeper relationship among all the excitement of a college campus. Patrick fell for her beautiful, big brown eyes and tall features. He was taken by her creativity as an interior design major, along with her determination and willingness to help others. When she visited our home, Fluffy enjoyed her delicate caressing. Best of all, Amy was willing to try *anything* I cooked. I wondered if she was just being polite, but she truly delighted in a broad spectrum of foods and flavors. They became college sweethearts.

Evan spent a month at home and then worked as a camp counselor. There is nothing like the responsibility of taking care of others to make you grow and stretch your insight. We enjoyed all of his camp stories, especially the stories about his second-grade campers insisting Evan was *old*. John and I reveled in his creative disciplinary skills when he made his camper count from one hundred to zero backward after hiding his bunkmate's socks and underwear. Evan was surrounded by the peace and power of the mountains and gained a new perspective and confidence to tackle his sophomore year of college. I was again unable to travel five hours away to move him into his new apartment. However, I did contribute by adding a mom's touch, purchasing and packing bedroom and kitchen items for his new pad.

Sarah's summer was filled with adventures at camp and on vacation. She immensely enjoyed time with her brothers at home, sleeping late, seeing her friends, and shopping online. Patrick plainly didn't understand why she needed more shoes! Sarah reached a major milestone, receiving her driver's permit and beginning a driving education course. Once she mastered parking lot driving, we ventured out of the neighborhood. She also babysat for our neighbors and worked in a community volunteer program. We were unable to participate in the mother-daughter charity league I had always expected we'd get to do together. Several weeks before school started, she made the high school volleyball team and began practices and games. Sarah looked forward to her sophomore year and was grateful the uncertainties of freshman year were behind her.

Our twenty-fifth wedding anniversary appeared. We felt compelled to celebrate in some grand fashion, especially since we weren't previously sure if we would reach our twenty-fourth anniversary the summer before. With my ongoing limitations, we learned to dial life's expectations down and find true value in the moment. Maybe being in the moment was the gift of chronic illness and the gift of being married twenty-five years. It was also the twenty-fifth anniversary of *The Lion King*, so we went to see the new movie version. Our date couldn't have been more appropriate. Our vow of "in sickness and in health" had begun with *The Lion King* love song twenty-five years earlier. We walked away inspired by the circle of life and the faith life demands. We spent several hours during this special week watching old family films of when we were all much younger. Now that was fun! I hadn't laughed so hard in a very long time. Watching our toddlers have a dance party in their pajamas with their cousins was wild to view again. They let loose in the foyer, flailing their little bodies left and right with abandon, then getting on the floor and kicking their feet in the air. It was so good for us to look back and remember a time when all was well.

Soon both boys were back at college, and I had renewed energy to take a leap. I drove myself an hour away to Sarah's volleyball tournament. I packed my salad for lunch, supplements, rose hip tea for my heart palpitations, and cooked vegetables for a snack, just in case I got stuck in traffic coming home. To the other parents, it was just another volleyball game. But to me, it was the first time that I'd gone out of town in months. Internally, I was doing a victory dance!

It had been a long time since I felt well enough to attend church, until one Sunday when the clouds lifted. I believe we receive what we need, somehow, at the perfect time we need it. During the service, a guest speaker was present, representing a mission house for the poor. This lovely lady educated the congregation about the needs of the people seeking their help. She spoke about the biblical parable of the lost son. In this story, the hard-working, obedient son grew angry when his disobedient brother returned home, asking for forgiveness after squandering all of his inheritance. The father welcomed him home with a celebration. Then he responded to the obedient son, "My son, you are here with me always; everything I have is yours," Luke 15:31. I'd heard the parable many times and had always focused on the message of forgiveness. The message of abundance, however, was hidden from me until that evening. Let those words sink in for a moment.

EVERYTHING I HAVE IS YOURS.

The lovely lady framed those words as what God tells each one of us, "Everything I have is yours!" She continued with, "No one is truly homeless because *our home is with God*. He meets all of our needs." I believe the speaker was saying that no matter what hardship you are experiencing, faith can have a huge impact. She said we all have a home with God in our hearts; it's always there, ready for us to tap into.

The parable is multifaceted, with tones of repentance, forgiveness, abundance, compassion, and dismissal of jealousy because we are all equal in His eyes. All this time I'd been trying to find my way.

I knew I wasn't home yet when the medical industry failed me. I was lost and where I didn't belong, so I turned to Jesus and to God for healing and to show me the way. I had been searching for my place of belonging and for answers to restore my health. I remembered so many Sundays, sitting in that very pew, with tears of desperation and hopelessness pouring down my cheeks, and my young daughter wiping them away. I was petrified of continuing to live with unbearable pain, and my mind was often filled with suicidal thoughts. I was aware of the stress it caused for my family and loved ones. I tried to be strong in public, yet in church I knew I couldn't hide my feelings anymore because He already knew.

The church hymns prompted me to finally release all my fears into His hands. I shed a layer of devastation amongst those colorful stained glass windows and burning candles. The Twilight Zone I had been living in vanished right there in church, as I thought to myself, *My search is over. I am home with God, and in His timeframe all the answers I have been in search of have been revealed.* Those answers were expertly and divinely delivered from above through Anthony William, the Medical Medium. I was finally free to move forward. I was free to celebrate the cures being the fruits, vegetables, leafy greens, herbs and spices, and wild foods that God has already provided for us all. Cures couldn't be found in labs or drugstores. Those were merely bandages. When you believe in God, you *see* God in everything, in everyone, in yourself, in every animal, in nature, and in every food. You see how we are all connected. When you realize that "everything He has is yours," then you realize *you have it all.*

New things, both large and small, began to pop up.

"Mom, can we please have the homecoming after-party at our house?" asked Sarah.

I quickly responded, "Sure!" The girls spent the night, and their dates left at 2:00 A.M. I woke up without any aftershocks.

That morning, as I sipped my lemon honey water, John blurted, "You *are* really getting better. You couldn't have tolerated hosting an after-party for Patrick and Evan's groups. Your supplements and foods *are* healing you!"

What? After almost three years of following Medical Medium, did John just say he *believed* I was healing? I had heard it myself, and I wished I had recorded it. I guess he'd finally seen a transformation in me. I had been showing him Instagram stories of people healing using Medical Medium information. The most convincing stories were the people covered in eczema and psoriasis who had taken all the medications on the market without success, then fully healed their gorgeous skin following Medical Medium protocols. They posted their before and after pictures, which were unmistakable. It was believing through sight.

I felt so well that I was able to stay for an entire varsity volleyball game, tolerating both the noise and excitement. I didn't return home until 9:00 P.M. and felt fine. I then dropped my evening supplement intake after six and a half years, except for the California poppyseed. I also had unexpected visits and calls from old friends out of the blue, and I could enjoy the camaraderie, relieved I was on the road to recovery.

John came with me to a writer's workshop in Houston, Texas. At the event, he pushed me around in a wheelchair to keep me off my feet and broken toes. I left the workshop extremely inspired to write. Originally, I had set up my office in Patrick's room, but soon all our kids were home, and demands grew while the globe moved through the COVID-19 pandemic. The kids attended school and college classes online, and John worked from home. Together, our worlds were unrecognizable; we learned so much about adapting and being flexible, and we had more time for self-reflection. After learning about the Lyme disease vaccine scandal, I was skeptical of the new vaccine everyone was being encouraged or forced to get. I remember everyone feeling captive, but it was a feeling to which I had grown accustomed. Patrick and Amy, along with their friends, were disappointed because they didn't have a formal graduation ceremony from college. I understood, but at the same time, I truly didn't have enough energy to travel. I didn't mind being home. It was my norm.

When it would be safe to come out again a year later, Amy and Patrick approached us, asking how we felt about having a July wedding in a short three months. Was it possible to plan a wedding and rehearsal dinner and whatever else had to be done in just three short months amid a pandemic? It would definitely be a quick turnaround, but we charged full steam ahead with wedding planning. Fortunately, Amy was decisive and knew what she liked. She already knew what she wanted in an engagement ring, and Patrick made it happen. He FaceTimed me from the jewelry store so I could be part of the selection process. The ring was created just in time for the engagement party that was held three-and-a-half hours away. As such, I had to move out of my comfort zone. The day after the party, we had lunch with Amy's parents, and the girls went across the street to a wedding dress boutique. Don't you know, Amy glowed with the first dress she tried on, and they had it altered in two weeks.

I didn't have the same luck, unfortunately. I was still three clothing sizes larger than my former comfortable size. My current weight literally felt heavy, yet I knew it was saving my life as my liver detoxed. I went shopping at a few stores to find a mother-of-the-groom dress. I bought one, even though it wasn't flattering on my papple shape. When I went to try it on again after the alterations, I stood in the dressing room quietly, weepy. It clearly wasn't how I wanted to look at my son's wedding. I told my friend, who encouraged me to keep shopping. Even though all I truly needed was a good attitude and smile on my face, I wanted to look somewhat put together. I tried one more nearby store and a fashionista angel put me in a long gown with a peplum covering my midsection—the papple. It was as good as any dress was going to get.

Sarah and I also needed clothing for the bridal shower and rehearsal dinner. My athleisure wardrobe perked up with colorful tops, white pants, shoes, dresses, and purses to match. Sarah, who always looks good in everything, was being selective, so we spent time outfitting her. John, Patrick, and Evan purchased new suits, shoes, and slacks. We were under a tight schedule and working hard, checking off our wedding to-do list. What I didn't expect was the emotional layer I had yet to address. I thought I had given Patrick full independence as he hadn't lived at home for five years.

When he walked in the door toward the end of the bridal shower, my maternal ears perked up. I heard him ask the hostess, "Where is she?" and I wanted to stand up and wave my arms and shout, "Here I am!" Then I saw a giant smile stretch across his face as he approached Amy, giving her a huge hug and kiss on her cheek. My heart felt knotted, giving a little tug when I quickly realized he'd been asking for his soon-to-be bride. A friend had given me some advice during that time, which proved to be an indispensable tool. She offered me some specific prayers incorporating everyone and all aspects revolving around a wedding. By reading them, I learned to move aside on my son's priority list and to open my heart wide to welcome the great blessing of a daughter-in-law. I learned to prayerfully ask God to make His face shine upon the new and permanent imprint of our growing and sacred family.

Before the big wedding weekend, other things began falling into place. Exercise became much easier for me. We went out and bought the last bike at the shop. Bike sales had climaxed during the pandemic since people were stuck at home. Riding my lime green bike, swimming laps, and going for walks were daily occurrences.

When my absent libido suddenly reappeared, whatever skepticism John had left of the Medical Medium information vanished. New and usable options of organic blush, foundation, mascara, and lipstick were quickly assembled in preparation for the big day. Organic eyeliners still caused me migraines, so they were avoided. Migraines were still an issue for me when using contacts, so I still had to wear my glasses. I missed how contacts kept my face free, but thank goodness the selection of glasses and sunglasses still remained plentiful.

After three years of cooking on my own, I hired Amber to help me prepare and cook food for the five days I'd be in a hotel for the wedding. We prepared salad fixings as we had done for Evan's competition. We also prepared four cooked vegetable dishes, which I ate for my dinners. The best part was Amber mentioning how much better I seemed physically and mentally. It was great to see her again, as we had previously spent a lot of time together. People were beginning to see the real me again.

I enjoyed personalizing all the details of the rehearsal dinner: the invitations, the champagne-colored tablecloths, and the tall, clear vases of blue and white hydrangea with roses and delphiniums. At each place setting were printed menus, place cards, and specially wrapped chocolates, while the beeswax candles added a hint of fresh air and ambiance. It felt like I was back in the saddle of my PTO days, where coordination never stopped. Prior to the rehearsal dinner, my food and our toaster oven were brought to the waitstaff. I was served with *my* food warmed and plated just like everyone else. *Oh, what a feeling!* Sarah had put together a slide show of the bride and groom, highlighting milestone moments with moving music. All attendees were very supportive of this couple, and the toasts were tremendously filled with so much love and friendship, elevating everyone in the room. The uplifted energy carried into the following day.

The stunning bride glided down the aisle on her father's arm with a knowing head tilt and modest smile as she watched Patrick wipe away his loving tears in anticipation. He was captivated by her. Her long, white, satin, Audrey Hepburn–style gloves sealed her elegance. Amy had always been a little girl who dreamed of her wedding day, and that dream was finally coming true! The figurative icing on the cake was my cousin's children as the flower girl and ring bearer. It was a time of uniting families in magnificent and upscale surroundings. A ten-piece band played, located under ten enormous chandeliers, illuminating the barely blue hints of color at the country club chosen for the reception. It was then that we had a special moment none of us will forget.

Amy's parents had hired a wonderful wedding planner who'd left nothing to chance. While the guests were escorted to a buffet-style feast, the parents and our children were escorted to a private room where we all ate dinner together. Again, I was served my food warm and plated, thanks to the insistence of Amy's mom. We had a chance to converse privately with our children as a newly married couple before sharing them with the other guests.

Oh, how I prayed for years to be the wife and mother I once was. I didn't want to miss any more monumental celebrations. I had prayed to be part of my children's weddings, and I finally was dancing with Patrick to "Shining Star" by *Earth, Wind & Fire*. We had only practiced the dance a few times, and my brain fog was still lifting. I was scared that I wouldn't remember the steps, so we wrote them down on a cheat sheet, and Evan knelt in front of the crowd and held it up for me. At this wedding, *I danced!* "Then young women will dance and be glad, young men and old as well. I will turn their mourning into gladness," Jeremiah 31:13.

For me, personally, the wedding was a declaration of wellness—a coming out of sorts, defying all the years I feared being wheelchair-bound. I had traveled, prepared, shopped, and planned wedding-related details as my heart expanded. I remained cautious, but I finally felt *alive*. The only hiccup was a migraine the morning of the wedding. But I slept it off and took what I needed to make it through the day. Amy and Patrick inspired me to let go of another layer of the past and merge deeper into life. They were so young and uninhibited with their can-do mindset. Seeing them chasing their dreams renewed my vigor to do the same.

The young couple had successfully planned a wedding in three months with their parents. Once married, they bought and moved into their first home. Amy managed a job change with a five-minute commute, then a goldendoodle puppy named Burleigh entered their lives. Naturally, one would expect a baby to follow that pattern. *Wait! A baby? Was I ready to be a grandmother—a hands-on grandmother?* I was resolved to keep rising to new life levels. I was motivated more than ever to stay on the Medical Medium wellness plan. Feeling more of my ailments drop away, along with the light within me burning brighter, was exactly how I wanted to meet my future grandchildren. It was how I wanted to celebrate Evan's college graduation and Sarah's high school graduation the following spring. It was how I wanted to start the empty nest adventure with John.

After the wedding, I found a penny in a grocery store parking lot. It wasn't a shiny, brand-new penny or a rusted, unrecognizable mess. It was simply a clean, warm, copper penny with experience that still held the promise of many tomorrows. I rarely found the pennies anymore, except when I needed to be reminded how "In God We Trust." Thank you, God, Anthony, and the Spirit of Compassion for the promise of more tomorrows. Thank you for making a way.

Weeks after the wedding, our family didn't escape the pandemic unscathed. My fully vaccinated dad was diagnosed with COVID pneumonia following a hurricane that had hit their town. The hurricane had prompted limited medical care, and multiple hospitals were out of service. After several unsuccessful visits to an alternate ER thirty minutes away, he was finally admitted to a room and sadly never returned home. I spent a month there with him. It was the first time that I'd driven six hours straight in nearly a decade. My mom and I took turns spending the days at the hospital, and I brought my food with me every time. At first, we thought he would recover. He was placed on a portable oxygen machine set to its maximum level. The goal was for the machine's oxygen level output to decrease, but it never did because my dad was dependent on the maximum amount. His X-rays showed complete scarring of his lungs. My dad had undiagnosed preexisting conditions with many symptoms, including weight loss. He looked in disgust under the hospital sheets at his skinny legs. He asked for a lung transplant but was told he wasn't a good candidate. We both realized the end was near for him, even though he was completely lucid. He had limited breath left.

I am so grateful for our time together because I missed him even before he was gone. I knew he didn't understand what I had been going through. Being consumed by my own sickness for so long, I had missed having normal time with him. During that month in the hospital, I learned a few things about my dad. I learned he had met my mom when she walked into his family music store looking for a job, and that my dad liked Elvis Presley's music. He told me, "I've had so many different kinds of experiences in my life." He felt his life had been full as he relived memories and said his parting words to loved ones over the phone.

It was gut-wrenching to watch him slip away. I asked friends who'd lost a parent if the shock of their absence ever left. Their general answer was a hard no. But it was my belief in a heaven full of unimaginable pleasure that helped me eventually find peace. I think I'll always miss his whistle, the sound of his voice, his presence, his nicknames for me, and the way he rubbed my back and called me baby doll. One of my dad's friends told my brother and me that our dad would be with us more than ever now. I feel him in so many ways daily, in words, in spirit, in pictures, and in our family.

Patrick once asked me what I had learned from my parents. I replied, "I learned to fight for myself and for the underdog from my dad, while my mom taught me I was loved and I was worthy." If you haven't been given these lessons, take them at this moment because you are worth fighting for, you are loved, and you are worthy of living a wonderful life!

During my dad's last month, my sister-in-law kept telling me how strong I was being. Honestly, I was surprised at my composure. I owed my grounding and stability, among the devastating trauma and loss, to the power of the living food I consumed. Food as medicine can be used for physical, mental, and emotional healing. I was so focused on physical healing that I had not realized the emotional and mental strength I'd gained on the journey until it had been put to the test. As hard as it was, I felt blessed to be there for my dad's departure from this Earth. A year earlier, I might not have been able to be there.

To my dad, I say, "You once told me somebody ought to do something. Writing this book is me doing something so someone else's son or daughter can heal." Matthew West has a song titled "Do Something," encouraging us to take a stand, to help others. I think to myself, *What if we all did something? What if we all followed our calling?* As Mother Teresa said, "There are no great acts, only small acts with great love."

Answers Known

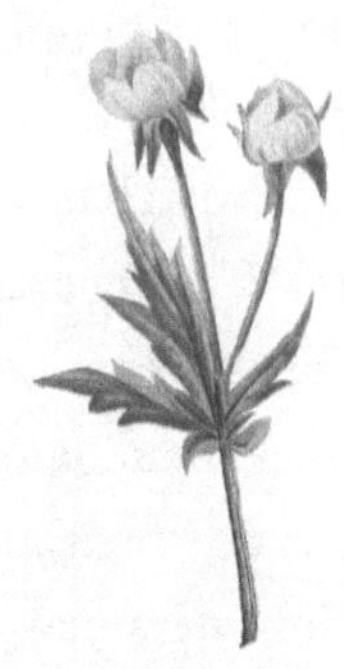

IN THIS BOOK, I'VE highlighted overcoming complex regional pain syndrome (CRPS), solanine toxicity syndrome, Lyme disease, and a slew of symptoms. But this isn't about me. It's so much bigger than me. This book contains my story, yet it is merely a reflection of others struggling with similar situations: going from doctor to doctor, taking part in one intervention after another, having relationship and family issues with no one believing or understanding their day-to-day backseat to life, and often facing financial distress. So, I scream from the rooftops, "ANSWERS HAVE BEEN FOUND!" Anthony William's Medical Medium book series has answers for many symptoms and conditions, even the big guns like addictions, attention-deficit/hyperactivity disorder (ADHD), amyotrophic lateral sclerosis (ALS), Alzheimer's disease, anxiety, arthritis, autism, cancer, depression, dementia, diabetes, gut issues, infertility, multiple sclerosis, neurological conditions, rheumatoid arthritis, and thyroiditis, and so on.

For example, in *Life-Changing Foods*, William says, "ninety-eight percent of the time, cancer is caused by an aggressive strain of a virus in combination with at least one kind of radical toxin." He offers a radio show found on SoundCloud titled "Cancer & Epstein Barr Virus," detailing what cancer really is, how it grows, and how to use food as medicine to battle it. Cancer is given this scary name with a big capital "C." My grandparents were so fearful of cancer, they wouldn't even mention the word. But what if it really has a viral pathogen element, with a lowercase "v"? I still dream of a world without cancer, without chronic illness. The Medical Medium book series offers new and poignant information for specific and general health questions alike. Some people might be confident and content with their care, while others have been on a lifelong search for *real* answers and *real* help to regain their lives. It's important for the general public to know they have choices in how to heal.

The year after my son's wedding and my dad's passing, we found a fresh start. The new home location we'd searched for years ago finally manifested. We sold our house, purchased another one, and remodeled it. We made it light and airy with lots of windows, white walls, and white oak floors. We placed shades of blues and greens throughout the home for a calming and restorative atmosphere. I love my new kitchen with its giant island and extra-wide sink. It's perfect for all the cooking we do and has plenty of space for our growing family. The new location suits us and our family's needs in a much better way, and it was great to shed the place reminding us of trauma and transformation. Joshua Radin's song "Brand New Day" was an ongoing prompt to leave the past in the past.

It was also a double graduation year. Evan graduated with a Bachelor of Science in finance and a Bachelor of Science in information systems and data science (ISDS) with a minor in analytics. He moved back to the Houston area and began a professional job for a global company using both of his degrees. Sarah graduated from high school and jumped into college life. She is studying to be a speech-language pathologist (SLP) with a focus on pediatrics and is about to transition from undergrad to graduate school. I was joyfully present for each of their relocations! Since we began the empty-nesting phase, I stopped cooking two different meals. John's reaction was to cook and eat with me and to cook other things for himself or eat out as he wished.

The following year, we were on the move. We took an adventurous family ski trip to Vail and a couple's trip to the U.S. Open Tennis Tournament in New York City. Both were a dream come true! In New York, we did touristy things, went to Broadway plays, and found a plant-based restaurant named abcV that was transparent with its ingredients, had a vast entrée assortment for me to choose from, and had a kind and knowledgeable waitstaff. We went several nights in a row! I still long to return because there are no restaurants in our area with such clean and delicious ingredients. We kept on moving. We moved Sarah into her college rental house, Evan into a condo, and my mom to Texas to reside near us.

When we were packing her things, her friends were discussing their various doctor appointments. One friend said, "When they've got you, they've got you." She was referring to the persistent doctor appointments, blood draws, scans, and tests intertwined into the fabric of their daily lives. I thought about how the Medical Medium information had set me free, and even though my journey was difficult, I am so grateful for finally being on this side of the mountain. I had been in a population I previously didn't know existed—the forgotten chronically ill. Now, I get to be the winner of my own life, and I don't live in constant fear of relapses or recurrence or of any other chronic illness making me dependent on big industries.

I remain grateful for each and every health professional who couldn't help me along the way because they encouraged me to keep searching. I continue to pray for the well-meaning health professionals who give of themselves daily, striving to assist patients to the best of their ability as they do phenomenal work. I learned that the health professionals weren't to blame. They simply have limitations because what they have been taught is limited and studies offer limited information. I'm grateful for the knowledge I've been empowered with to raise myself out of bed and back into life. From the Medical Medium series, I'd found the equal and opposite reaction to return to health. I'm so grateful because 2023 was the year we welcomed our first granddaughter into the world.

We were all there for Brooke's birth. I was her first babysitter. I encouraged Amy and Patrick to ride together to pick up their dinner while I sat holding Brooke in the rocking chair. I studied her tiny little fingers and her tiny little toes, just the two of us in their quiet, cozy home. I swayed in amazement at my baby having a baby as I snuggled her closely. I kept thinking, *We get to keep her! She is ours!* Shopping for baby clothes again became my sweetest delight, and experiencing all the newborn firsts again filled me with wonder. I was able to dive into the blessings of grandparenthood with sheer joy!

Life just kept getting better and better, and I kept rising to it. I weaned off the California poppyseed pain supplement, but I continue to take Medical Medium maintenance supplements. I use food as medicine per the book's protocols, bake and cook with John, often trying new recipes, and remain off prescription medications. William teaches that sleep can be recouped once we've done enough healing. These days I've been sleeping eight to ten hours a night, and my body temperature has regulated. I'm no longer anemic, no longer cold all the time, and enjoying casual tennis dates!

In January of 2024, John and I went on a ski trip to Beaver Creek, Colorado. It was only the two of us, and it was amazing! We skied a lot since the slopes were vacant. Nothing was holding us back! In the spring, we hosted a wedding shower for one of Patrick's high school best friends. It was a rainy day, but the adorable couple didn't care as they enjoyed all the festivities, gifts, food, and games. We also hosted a brunch and wedding prep day for my cousin's daughter and her wedding party. I had fresh flowers and tablecloths placed on the tables. She was a blissful bride, basking in the support from friends and family members, and glowing from the love of her fiancé. After the wedding, John assisted with taking down the decorations late into the night. The next morning, I walked into our kitchen and living room and was taken aback because the flowers had multiplied. There were big, bright, beautiful flowers *everywhere*. I thought back about the prayers spoken over me at the ladies' gym about flowers blooming in the desert. I knew the dreary desert times were gone, and there in my kitchen, those big, bright, beautiful blossoms found me. I had *bloomed*, and our new landscaping and garden had bloomed as well.

There were more adventures to be had! We took the whole family to the beach for a week at the beginning of the summer. I went to the beach each day, and we played charades during the afternoon rain showers. We laughed, cooked, played games, and watched movies. It was the first beach trip where I didn't take a single pain pill or supplement, where I didn't miss a thing, and where John didn't have the stress of work on his mind. For our thirtieth wedding anniversary, John and I visited West Palm Beach. We ate at another fantastic restaurant called Christopher's Kitchen that had the Heavy Metal Detox Smoothie on its menu! They also customized dishes for Medical Medium compliance. I'm talking about the best gluten-free, plant-based pizza I've ever tasted, with whipped macadamia nut cheese and more! I long to return there as well.

Our actual anniversary day was full. The morning began with water aerobics in the hotel's infinity pool overlooking the Atlantic Ocean. Nora, our instructor, embodied her dancing history with her long, lean legs, rhythm, and athletic disposition. Besides her outgoing personality, her tunes were inspiring, as we kicked and bounced, singing about believing in miracles.

Our day continued with massages and then dinner at Christopher's Kitchen, followed by salsa dancing lessons. The class was filled with men and women half our age, but we gave it a carefree whirl, because why not! We had much to celebrate. Prior to flying home, we gave Nora the blender we'd bought there for our stay. She reported that she uses the blender each morning to make herself a fruit smoothie. She's got the right idea!

As fall approached, John's company merged with another, and he chose not to stay on board. Instead, he took a step back and said he wanted to cook our dinners so I could finish writing this book. He gave me room for no more excuses. It's interesting what happens when one door closes. The day after he finished his job, we headed to Los Angeles and were able to secure tickets to a Medical Medium pop-up dinner at Café Gratitude. We got to meet Anthony William in person!

I was a mess that day. I was extremely and unusually nervous. I'd learned not to place people on pedestals, since it gives them a platform from which to fall. But come on, this guy was my hero! I tried to picture meeting him. I wanted to be calm and collected. I didn't know what I'd say though, and everything was being filmed. I'd probably only have a couple of minutes, although I wished for a couple of hours—as everyone else did in line. I wrote him a thank-you card in case I couldn't come up with the right words. I wanted to be relaxed, but I had waited eight years for this moment. As we stepped toward him on the red carpet, the first thing I noticed was his luminous skin that was so perfect and creamy.

I excitedly blurted out, "You *saved* my life; you *saved* our marriage!" So much for playing it cool. I was a tense groupie.

He focused in on John, asking, "So, who is this strapping guy?" He was laughing and shaking John's hand. He was careful to point out the spouses because many spouses were insecure and not supportive of the Medical Medium lifestyle.

John took the opportunity to extend his appreciation, replying, "I want to thank you for giving me my wife back."

William kept his hand on my shoulder, likely sending me healing energy. I became much more lighthearted. Then he placed his other hand on John's shoulder, encircling the three of us.

"You two are meant to be together," he revealed.

Earlier that day, John asked me what my expectations were of meeting Anthony William. I tried not to have any, but I mentioned I'd like some kind of takeaway from the experience. Even though meeting him was brief, it's something I'll never forget. That night, we walked into Café Gratitude and had to find a table. There was a table of four ladies with two open seats on the patio, which is where we landed. The lady sitting next to me was from Dallas, and sitting next to her was her friend from Austin. We all bonded over living in Texas. The other two ladies were from Hawaii and Nevada. The four of them had shared an Airbnb for the weekend.

Over dinner, we told our stories and ate the most delicious and nutritious food. The lady from Hawaii was a very spiritual yoga instructor and was drawn to the truth of the Medical Medium series, striving to live her best life. The lady from Nevada battled Lyme disease and had come a long way and now was a social butterfly with the most compassionate heart. The lady from Dallas used the Medical Medium series to heal herself from a life of addiction and now works with others struggling with addictions. Talk about paying it forward! The lady from Austin was the leader of the Austin Medical Medium group, which meets monthly for meals and outings. She incredibly healed herself from ALS beginning symptoms using the book series' information, curing the incurable! She gave me the cellphone number of the Medical Medium group leader in Houston. Right then and there, I joined a Medical Medium group in our hometown. Now, we meet monthly for potluck dinners and friendship, a larger takeaway than I'd ever imagined. My tribe is growing! We met an entire community of Medical Medium followers who've been on their own healing journeys. I was amazed to see people from other countries using their time and resources to travel and be a part of this global movement. There were even young couples who brought their babies and children to the event to thank Anthony William for helping them achieve their fertility goals.

While in Los Angeles, we hit all the spots, and John took a surfing lesson. Despite the twenty-five-year-old surf instructor's warning that most people our age couldn't get on the board, John did it! Who knows what we'll do next or where we will go? Café Gratitude and Berbere are two LA restaurants I definitely long to return to.

Our children were super impressed with John's ability to surf. They've witnessed my resurrection, and each in their own way has benefited from all I've learned. Patrick and Amy found a holistic pediatrician. They use many of the Medical Medium tools to treat Brooke with minor symptoms. Amy has even helped a friend clear her baby's respiratory infection using its suggestions. She used some of William's ideas for her pregnancies to prevent postpartum depression and to help her breast milk be plentiful. She even had extra breast milk to donate.

Evan was able to stay out of the hospital when his chest X-ray indicated pneumonia. Although his X-ray showed a severe case of pneumonia, he wasn't in severe respiratory distress and his oxygen saturation was normal. I used the Medical Medium recommendations with him, and Evan combined them with his prescription antibiotic. It took several weeks, but his lungs completely cleared.

One day out of the blue, Sarah surprised me with a texted photo of her very own celery juice that she'd picked up from a nearby juice bar. She said it made her feel really good, and she continued to purchase more.

Now, each of our children has their own set of Medical Medium–recommended supplements to use as they choose, whether as a preventative or to treat illness as it comes. In addition, they all ask me to help them with assorted health-related issues. They each have an in-depth understanding that everyone is going through something, and they value compassion more than ever. Will they one day take a deeper dive into the benefits of the Medical Medium protocols? That decision is for them to decide on their own time frame. They each have their own path and their own lessons to learn. What I do know is that life includes difficult times, and life is easier when you believe in yourself, when you believe in something greater than yourself, and when you embody good health.

I knew before this manuscript went to print that there was one more stop I needed to make. I returned to my primary caregiver and asked for an EBV blood test. I explained what I'd been doing and what I needed to the nurse practitioner. She was intrigued. I mentioned, "I know you have patients with symptoms you can't help."

She replied, "Yes, and it is frustrating!"

"Check out the Medical Medium series of books, which are written like medical textbooks. They are expanding on the educational foundation of health professionals and assisting them to help their patients," I remarked.

My EBV result was a whopping *zero*. The test prior to using the Medical Medium protocols was 103, with a normal range being 0.0–17.9. At first glance, my blood test seemed to reveal quite a success story. I already knew I'd found success, however, because I was finally living my life again. This EBV test, known as a polymerase chain reaction (PCR), is meant to find the DNA of EBV in the bloodstream upon an initial infection. What I'd forgotten was that EBV doesn't stick around in the blood to be found. As William wrote, in time, EBV *conceals* itself in our organs and nervous system. So, it's safe to say, currently, there are no valid medical tests to determine a chronic case of the virus. Nor are there current valid medical tests for the other Unforgiving Six: dichlorodiphenyltrichloroethane (DDT) and other applications, radiation, adrenaline triggers, civil sabotage, and heavy metals. It makes me even more grateful for the work of the Medical Medium series and the Spirit of Compassion and for the Holy Five (fruits, vegetables, leafy greens, herbs and spices, and wild foods).

At the end of the most recent Medical Medium podcasts, a recording states that the Medical Medium information has never been proven wrong by medical science and research, only proven right. It encourages people to cite where their information comes from if they use original published Medical Medium information because it's often stolen and used by others in their practices and on social media. Citation is important because it enables people to locate the books for use, so they can receive their full and unmatched benefits to a healthy life, like I did. In retrospect, I received tidbits of Medical Medium information from an Austin physician, but she never cited the information or explained it convincingly. Perhaps this information was new to her, but maybe I would have healed quicker if I could've located it faster.

To the reader, I appreciate you, and I want you to know that I'm praying for your healing and the healing of your loved ones. I really am. Maybe you don't need a complete Medical Medium overhaul like I did. Maybe you just need some help to release toxins or to weed out an old habit or addiction. Maybe like a starved plant, you simply need new soil with new nutrients. Perhaps you need Medical Medium meditations, cleanses, or therapies to bloom. Suppose you just need to prune or cut out some of the troublemaker foods to find your answer. Whatever you need, rest assured that the most profound healing tools on the planet are now within your reach. I hope you'll find big, bright, beautiful flowers of your own. The next chapter for John and myself has already started, with the birth of our first grandson, Jack. There are now more little baby clothes, more tiny little fingers and tiny little toes, more firsts, and much more wonder. God be with you!

"See, I am doing a new thing! Now it springs up; do you not perceive it? I am making a way in the desert and streams in the wasteland." Isaiah 43:19 from *Jesus Today*.

View from a Spouse

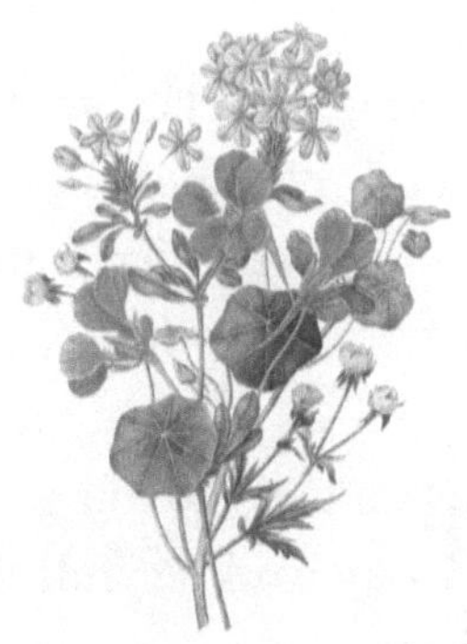

"THE BEST IS YET TO BE." Deborah had these words inscribed inside a new wedding band she gave me for our twenty-seventh wedding anniversary. We were seven years into our healing journey. The words not only represented exciting times ahead, but they also showed me the future she saw in *us*. During the journey, however, I never would have imagined these six words would've been said between us.

As Deborah's spouse, I was called to write and share this chapter for those spouses and caregivers who are as uncertain of their futures as the person who is sick. You might not be the one who is sick or the one everyone is asking about, but you'll still feel much of the same anger, frustration, confusion, and anxiety. My hope is that reading this chapter and seeing Deborah's journey through my eyes, coupled with four life lessons, provides some understanding and encouragement of the path on which you're walking. Your part in this healing process isn't only vitally important to the physical healing taking place, it can also lead to healthier, stronger relationships and great times ahead.

As with many of life's unexpected events, it all began pretty easily.

When Deborah first injured her wrists, we were thinking it would be a simple fix. Broken bones and sprained ligaments are common, everyday accidents that happen to many people. Doctors place them in a cast or splint, then you add a little therapy, and you're good as new. My role while she healed was to take care of her and all the things she did for our family. Before her fall, I was working full-time while Deborah stayed home taking care of our three children. After her fall, I backed off from work for a bit and began helping around the house. With both her wrists immobile, she needed help with everything from brushing her hair to getting dressed. On my way home from work, I would pick up groceries from the store, then heat up dinner that Amber had prepared for us. I also helped our kids with their homework and school projects and often drove the daily carpools to school and practices. All these efforts helped her focus on her healing quickly so our lives could return to normal. That's how it had always been. Why should this have been any different? However, when the term "complex regional pain syndrome" was mentioned by her doctors and nurses, it became very real that this was not going to be a quick fix.

Things became more confusing and frustrating as we moved deeper into the unknown causes of her pain. Not only was she *not* getting better, but she was actually getting worse. She was in constant pain and always fatigued, which kept her bedridden most days. When she was upright, she spent time on the computer, searching for any answers about why she was sick and how to heal. Many of our friends and family had started to notice she was continuing to suffer. Some just stopped calling as their lives got busy, and some continued to call but were as confused as we were. Others called me privately, offering suggestions of doctors to see, treatments to try, or mental therapies to incorporate. The more research Deborah did, however, the more her symptoms pointed to CRPS, which causes intense chronic pain with no known cure. The only medical course of action offered was cervical nerve blocks to block her pain, followed by intense therapy.

I was so scared and angry that this was happening to *us*. We'd had such a wonderful life up to that point, with healthy kids, a beautiful home, and a good job. We were doing all the things doctors and alternative practitioners had recommended us to do. It was always *try this medication or that supplement. Do more therapy. Eat this, not that.* Yet nothing was working. And during our research, we found that, in some cases, patients with CRPS even committed suicide just to make their pain go away. The thought of Deborah wanting to take her own life was so hard for me to wrap my brain around. But, as I later found out, at times, that was exactly where she was!

As the years went by, I felt Deborah and I pulling apart as a couple while we dealt with what was happening. She was focused on handling her pain and researching treatments, while I was focused on hurrying the process along so we could return to normal. We were so preoccupied that we didn't *see* each other. At one point, we actually had an intense shouting match in our backyard, and I began yelling, "I am doing all I can do! What else do you want me to do?"

You see, as a husband, I always thought that one of my jobs was to *fix* things. If a light was out, I changed the bulb. If the brakes on our car needed changing, I brought it to the mechanic's shop. With Deborah's illness, I figured if I picked up the slack with the family, allowed her the time to heal, and supported her through her struggles, then all would get better. I was doing all I could for her so she could get healthy. That's when my first life lesson of our health journey occurred: In that shouting match, Deborah yelled back at me, "This is not about you!" And she was right!

During all that time, I had become so focused on how *I* could help her. What could *I* do so that *my* world could return back to normal? I had always heard about unconditional love but never knew what that meant until now. The dictionary defines it as love without conditions. The condition I was living out was placing all my efforts in her healing so *I* could be happy again. When you get married and say, "in sickness and in health, for better or for worse," everyone thinks about the healthy and better days. Well, this was one of those "sickness" and "worse" times where unconditional love was tested. In that moment, I made a decision to change my mental state and frame of mind and to focus on Deborah, her healing, and our family. It became less about the future I had in my mind and more about the day-to-day and being present. So, I did, or at least tried, my best.

Our healing journey moved deeper into the unknown. Over time, her injured wrists did show signs of healing, but she was still in constant pain and chronically fatigued. She saw cardiologists, pain specialists, orthopedists, hematologists, and therapists. Her symptoms continued, and it was clear and depressing that modern medicine could not help. At our ropes' end, we began researching alternative practices and came across a chiropractor in the mountains who used holistic methods to treat patients. With a glimmer of hope that he might be able to do what no other doctor could do, we scheduled an appointment and flew out to see him. It was there that he diagnosed Deborah with Lyme disease.

Now, Lyme disease is a terrible illness in itself. If you read about it, people suffer for life in some cases. But for us, it was a bit of a relief. We finally had an answer and something we could look to treat. Since traditional medicine had failed us before, we switched to holistic practitioners and methods to treat Lyme disease. Some methods were pretty radical and required a lot of faith, but that was where we were in our journey. We were trying anything and everything that gave us hope she could heal. I muscle-tested her three times a day to get what we thought was the right supplement combination. We bought an infrared sauna and placed it in our garage so she could use it three times a week to detox. We used a Rife machine to try and kill pathogens with ultrasonic frequencies. We even tried bee venom therapy, which required me to place live bees on her back so they would sting her. All these things were done with the hope of finding The One that would cure her and give us our lives back. But one after the other, these practices did not heal Deborah. She continued to suffer and remained fatigued. And I became angrier and more frustrated. I started to believe we were on a never-ending journey and doubted any remedies could be found for her illness.

Then a book was suggested to Deborah that was written by Anthony William, known as the Medical Medium. He basically focuses on the Epstein-Barr virus and other herpes viruses being the root cause of numerous illnesses. He encourages taking specific supplements and eating fruits, leafy greens, vegetables, herbs and spices, and wild foods (known as the Holy Five) to aid in the healing process. He also stresses the belief in the body's ability to heal itself.

At first, I approached Mr. William's protocols with much doubt. To me, they were just another thing added to a long line of failed treatments for healing. I didn't want to get too invested in them since, like the others, we likely would be onto another therapy or protocol soon. Equally as frustrating, however, was the fact the protocols weren't simply a healing technique; it was a whole lifestyle change. The protocol called for Deborah to change her eating habits further, in addition to eliminating any toxins and virus-feeding foods. It meant preparing *all* her meals at home to manage exactly what food she was eating and how it was prepared. No longer could we enjoy dinners out with friends, and picking up takeout wasn't an option for Deborah. Meals had to be prepared ahead of time and packed whenever we traveled. I resisted all these changes and tried to cope by telling myself *she* was healing, not me. Dinners consisted of

Deborah cooking two different meals, one for herself and one for the rest of the family. This regulated and separated lifestyle made us drift even further apart as a married couple. It finally reached a really dark stage when we planned our summer trip to Breckenridge.

We had previously taken family trips to Colorado in the wintertime, but we'd never visited during the summer. All of our kids are athletic and enjoy the outdoors, so we thought it would be fun to experience the mountains in the summertime. Deborah knew that her restrictions and physical condition would hinder our activities, but I wanted to go and have a little mountain getaway from our day-to-day lives. So, we both decided she would stay home, and I would take the kids. As we were leaving, I knew it was a mistake to leave her behind and felt a huge hole in my heart that she wasn't with us. Not having my best friend next to me to experience the funny moments and beautiful scenery of our trip tore me apart. The fact that we both decided her remaining behind was the best answer for the two of us and our family was even more depressing.

Through my anger and frustration, along with Deborah feeling stranded to face this monster alone without my support, our marriage began to really break down. We weren't on the same page about most things, and instead of talking and communicating, we simply shut each other out. All of the affection, hugs, kisses, "good-nights," and "I love yous" that couples with healthy, happy marriages have had faded away. We became distant—just two people passing each other day and night. Deep down we knew we still loved each other, so we decided to reach out to a therapist.

Through therapy and counseling, I learned my second life lesson: *All relationships change and transform into something different every day.* For me, Deborah started out as my girlfriend, then my wife, then the mother of our children, and now an empty nester and grandmother. All these roles required her and our relationship to evolve for it to continue to work. While reflecting back on over thirty-five years of being in a relationship together, my third life lesson came shining in: *I had changed along the way with her.* I just never realized it. I had evolved from the man I was to the man I was becoming. We had transformed and recreated the love we had for each other in each phase. According to our therapist, each phase offered two choices:

1. Do I want to make the transformation?
2. Do I want to stay in this relationship?

For me, it was decision time. Did I want to change bits and pieces of my lifestyle and fully support Deborah with the Medical Medium guidance and direction being the answer? And was Deborah the one I wanted to spend the golden years of my life with? After much praying, my answer to both questions was a resounding *YES!*

I decided to learn more about the Medical Medium protocols so we could walk this journey together. I learned about the benefits of taking daily supplements, eating fresh fruits and vegetables, and how our bodies can heal themselves over time. I learned that everything we put into our bodies, as well as everything within our environment, plays a part in our health. The more I read and learned, the more I became convinced that the

Medical Medium protocols would not only help Deborah but could help me as well. I began going to the grocery store and buying organic vegetables and fruits. I cut back on eating meat, had smoothies for breakfast and salads for lunch, and helped Deborah cook organic, plant-based meals for dinner. While I definitely didn't follow the protocol rigidly, I did improve what I was eating and began taking supplements.

Many people see immediate results when they start eating better. For Deborah and me, it was a slow and gradual process. Along the way, I found we were becoming less and less frustrated and angry with each other. We started to connect more and enjoyed each other's company. I actually enjoyed cooking, to the total surprise of my family. As the years went by, she started to feel better day by day. The Medical Medium protocol was working, was very simple, and offered my fourth life lesson: *What you eat matters. How you treat yourself matters. And your body can heal itself.*

The challenging part of this new lifestyle was dealing with society. It is very hard to find a restaurant that serves healthy foods with clean ingredients. However, most social settings are scheduled around either eating out or meeting for drinks. So, we adapted as best we could. We invited people to our house to visit or went to their house to catch up. When we did eat out, Deborah would eat at home ahead of time. Knowing we were on this journey together, side by side, made coming home to her after work the best part of my day.

As time passed, I actually began to feel better. I noticed I had more energy, could run farther at the gym, and returned to the weight I was in my thirties. Even my doctors could see the difference. When I was in my early forties, I was diagnosed with hemochromatosis (an iron-overload condition—the opposite of anemia). I had to give blood every three months as part of a protocol called phlebotomies to keep my iron levels down. My liver specialist, a hepatologist, told me no pill or diet could lower my iron to manageable levels, and that phlebotomies were the only answer. Since I was feeling better, I decided to stop going to the blood bank and try letting my Medical Medium protocol do the trick. After two years, I revisited my doctor to get my annual phlebotomy prescription renewed, and miraculously, my levels were normal. So normal, in fact, that the doctor didn't even prescribe the phlebotomies anymore.

Currently, we continue to use the Medical Medium protocols and view ourselves as living proof of what it can do. Deborah has gone from being bedridden to skiing down the Colorado slopes with our family. We have traveled all over the country and are excited about the new adventures lying ahead. I feel wonderful, with normal blood levels resulting from what I eat instead of from taking cholesterol and blood pressure medications. We recently celebrated our thirtieth wedding anniversary, recognizing the journey we have been through and the growing love we continue to build.

Miracles definitely come in all different shapes and sizes. For Deborah and me, it started with a book by Anthony William that changed our lives and placed us on a track that neither of us could've predicted fifteen years ago. It's a track that has brought us closer together as a couple, strengthening not only our relationship but our bodies.

To all the spouses and caregivers reading this book, know that this journey is not all about *you*. But *you* do need to walk the path of a supporting and loving partner for real healing to occur in your partner's life. Know that the couple you are today will never be the couple you were yesterday. However, the couple you will be tomorrow will have adventures of their own. And know that this journey won't only lead to better health for your partner, it can lead to better health for you as well. I pray this book brings you some hope that, as hard as the journey seems, "The Best is Yet to Be."

References

Basilio, Humberto. "'Mono' Virus May Also Cause Lupus." *scientificamerian.com*. November 12, 2025. www.scientificamerican.com/article/the-epstein-barr-virus-may-cause-lupus.

Bean, Constance A. and Lesley Ann Fein. *Beating Lyme: Understanding and Treating This Complex and Often Misdiagnosed Disease*. AMACOM, 2008.

Holy Bible, New International Version. Biblica, 2011.

Johnson, Lorraine. "LYMEPOLICYWONK: Pam Weintraub's CNN Article—Setting Things Straight." *lymedisease.org*. July 13, 2013. www.lymedisease.org/lymepolicywonk-pam-weintraubs-cnn-article-setting-things-straight-3/.

New American Bible, Saint Joseph Edition. Catholic Book Publishing Company, 1992.

Shanley, Deborah M. "Special Report: American Medical Association is Injuring Patients with RSD." International Research Foundation for RDS/CRPS. July 20, 2020. www.rsdfoundation.org/test/AMA.html.

The Holy Bible, English Standard Version. Crossway, 2001.

Watson, Stephanie. "Vitamins and Supplements: How to Choose Wisely." *WebMD*. August 7, 2025. www.webmd.com/diet/how-to-evaluate-vitamins-supplements.

Weintraub, Pamela. *Cure Unknown: Inside the Lyme Epidemic, Revised Edition*. St. Martin's Griffin, 2013.

Weintraub, Pamela. "Why You Should Be Afraid of Lyme Disease." *CNN*. July 29, 2013. www.cnn.com/2013/07/12/opinion/weintraub-lyme-disease.

William, Anthony, host. *Radio Show Archive by Medical Medium*. "Cancer & Epstein Barr Virus." SoundCloud, November 3, 2017. Podcast, 1:55:25. https://soundcloud.com/medicalmedium/cancer-epstein-barr-virus.

William, Anthony. *Medical Medium: Secrets Behind Chronic and Mystery Illness and How to Finally Heal, Revised and Expanded Edition*. Hay House, 2021.

William, Anthony. *Medical Medium Brain Saver: Answers to Brain Inflammation, Mental Health, OCD, Brain Fog, Neurological Symptoms, Addiction, Anxiety, Depression, Heavy Metals, Epstein-Barr Virus, Seizures, Lyme, ADHD, Alzheimer's, Autoimmune & Eating Disorders*. Hay House, 2022.

William, Anthony. *Medical Medium Brain Saver Protocols, Cleanses & Recipes : For Neurological, Autoimmune & Mental Health*. Hay House, 2022.

William, Anthony. *Medical Medium Celery Juice: The Most Powerful Medicine of Our Time Healing Millions Worldwide*. Hay House, 2019.

William, Anthony. *Medical Medium Cleanse to Heal: Healing Plans for Sufferers of Anxiety, Depression, Acne, Eczema, Lyme, Gut Problems, Brain Fog, Weight Issues, Migraines, Bloating, Vertigo, Psoriasis, Cysts, Fatigue, PCOS, Fibroids, UTI, Endometriosis & Autoimmune.* Hay House, 2020.

William, Anthony. *Medical Medium Life-Changing Foods: Save Yourself & Your Loved Ones With Fruits, Leafy Greens, Herbs, Wild Foods & Vegetables, Expanded Edition.* Hay House, 2025.

William, Anthony. *Medical Medium Liver Rescue: Answers to Eczema, Psoriasis, Diabetes, Strep, Acne, Gout, Bloating, Gallstones, Adrenal Stress, Fatigue, Fatty Liver, Weight Issues, SIBO & Autoimmune Disease.* Hay House, 2018.

William, Anthony. *Medical Medium Thyroid Healing: The Truth Behind Hashimoto's, Graves', Insomnia, Hypothyroidism, Thyroid Nodules & Epstein-Barr.* Hay House, 2017.

William, Anthony, host. *Radio Show Archive by Medical Medium.* "Truth about Protein." SoundCloud, 2019. Podcast, 54:53. https://soundcloud.com/medicalmedium/truth-about-protein.

William, Anthony, host. *Radio Show Archive by Medical Medium.* "Truth about Multiple Sclerosis." SoundCloud, May 16, 2017. Podcast, 54:51. https://soundcloud.com/medicalmedium/truth-about-multiple-sclerosis?in=brow-zing/sets/medmead.

Young, Sarah. *Jesus Calling: Enjoying Peace in His Presence, A 365-Day Devotional.* Thomas Nelson, 2004.

Young, Sarah. *Jesus Today: Experience Hope Through His Presence, A 150-Day Devotional.* Thomas Nelson, 2012.

Acknowledgments

First, I thank God for this rocky road and expansive growth I have experienced, and for never letting me go. I see now how You can use our story to help others, and I see how this story is so much bigger than me!

Second, I thank Anthony William for his courage to accept such a unique role in global healing. Without you and your work with the Spirit of Compassion, I don't know if I'd still be alive or have any quality of life, and I know others feel the same way. This work of yours is the greatest miracle of our time! I respect and admire you wholeheartedly.

To Muneeza, thank you for your passion and persistence in teaching us how to best use the Medical Medium tools to heal. It was your belief in healing that sparked mine.

Anne and Cindy, you gave me a sisterhood of belonging and acceptance that I will always treasure.

To my family, thank you all for joining me on this wild and confusing journey, for delving into these uncharted waters by my side. You've each pushed me, encouraged me, and motivated me to make space for a new way of life. You all are the reasons I fought so hard to stay here and heal, and I'm so glad I did. I love you more than you know.

To my husband, thank you for all the smoothies in bed, the muscle testing, the bee stings, and for the support during the years of uncertainty. Thank you for teaching me that we all grow and accept change on our own timeline. It feels really good to start a new journey with you by my side. The best is yet to be!

To my friends old and new, I'm very ready to connect on a deeper level now that this book is complete. I have missed you. How about a smoothie? I know Dr. Phan wants one! Hats off to Dr. Phan, who is one of many doctors on the forefront, tirelessly getting the Medical Medium information out to their patients. You are doing God's work.

To the late Nancy Whisenhunt and her sister, Ginny Strath-dee, thank you from the bottom of my heart for your care and concern, and for telling my mom about the Medical Medium book. Because of your kindness, I am well, and hopefully this book will encourage others to find wellness, all because you spoke up.

To Natalie, thank you for being there through the years as a steady and longtime trusted friend. Thank you for the calls, the walks, the listening, the problem-solving and even bee stings when John was unavailable.

To each person mentioned in the book, thank you for playing your part to move my story along. You are a reminder of community being essential, that we are never alone, and that sometimes it takes a village.

To KN Literary Arts, thank you for your services in pulling this book together in readable form. I believe the people you have placed in our life to help us along the way were meant to be. Carolyn Flynn, Jennifer Holder, Janette Lynn, Elisabeth Rinaldi, Erin Seaward-Hiatt, Audra Figgins, and Grainne Daly: Together, you all have extracted a creative side in me to write scenes, organize paragraphs, edit pages, and picture a book cover. I've enjoyed being your pupil and have a much greater appreciation for the literary world. The readers can thank you all for a beautiful, well-organized and professional book.

To the reader, thank you for your support, and I hope you've received a takeaway from my manuscript. God bless you on your own healing journey. May we all work together for a healthier world.

About the Author

Deborah Kelly is a former oncology nurse, former stay-at-home mom, and now an empty nester. After overcoming a decade of chronic illness, her purpose is to offer understanding, hope, and faith in healing. She and her husband are the proud parents of three children, a daughter-in-law, and two grandchildren. You may find them cooking, exercising, gardening, and traveling, when not spending time with their friends and family. Deborah is an avid advocate for wellness and healing with the Medical Medium information.

To contact Deborah, email her at makingawayrising@gmail.com.

She and her husband, John, plan to donate a portion of the book proceeds to organizations dedicated to helping others heal by using Medical Medium tools.

www.ingramcontent.com/pod-product-compliance
Lightning Source LLC
Chambersburg PA
CBHW020335180726
47991CB00020B/1703